THE

Parasite
Menace

THE
Parasite
MENACE

SKYE WEINTRAUB, N.D.

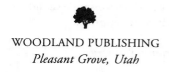

WOODLAND PUBLISHING
Pleasant Grove, Utah

©1998
Woodland Publishing
P.O. Box 160
Pleasant Grove, UT
84062

Printed in the United States of America

Contents

Foreword

I recently met Dr. Weintraub through mutual friends who knew that we were both writing books on parasites. When I saw her book, I discovered that she had included almost everything I wanted to say and a lot more. I decided to stop writing my book for now and concentrate on the next step. This is making the public aware of the parasite problem and stimulating research in this area. We need facts to stimulate research and we need research to convince health care professionals about the enormity of parasitic infections. Dr. Weintraub will help greatly to create public awareness of parasites and provide a variety of approaches to treat these infections.

My experience with parasites goes back 40 years when I studied about parasites at the London School of Hygiene and Tropical Medicine. For two years I was a government medical officer in Tanzania, East Africa, where every patient I saw had at least three parasites. In spite of my great knowledge and experience with parasites in Africa, I was like the rest of the doctors in North America. I believed that parasites were only a major problem in tropical third-world countries.

My opinion changed when my patients and others began seeing many worms, flukes, and other visible parasites in their stools after treatment. After passing worms, many chronic health conditions improved greatly. I know that two thirds of the parasites are microscopic so that these findings indicated that parasitic infections may be very common. Next, I heard about several people with biopsy-proven cancer passing worms. I was amazed and wondered if there could be a connection. Were parasites a cofactor in the causation of cancer? Were they making cancers worse by weakening the immune system?

In *The Parasite Menace,* Dr. Weintraub explains why there may be a connection between parasites and chronic diseases. She presents a compelling case that many people have parasites and that this problem is rapidly increasing. This book should be a great stimulus to create public interest about a neglected topic. I believe it is of great importance to learn more about parasites.

I particularly like Dr. Weintraub's discussion of toxicity and detoxification. She provides sound reasons as to how we have become increasingly exposed to internal and external toxins, but that our ability to eliminate these toxins from our bodies have become impaired. Even my colleagues in mainstream medicine will surely agree that normal metabolism produces waste products that must be excreted through the kidneys, liver, lungs, skin and bowel. The most important of these excretory organs is the bowel. Yet there is good evidence that at least 80 percent of us are relatively constipated and therefore unable to adequately get rid of waste products.

It is important to understand how necessary it is to have good bowel health and to make toxicity a top priority. If I were doing research today, I would concentrate on getting the facts about parasites to the public. *The Parasite Menace* is a provoking book that I hope will be read by medical students and doctors, as well as the general public.

DR. F. RUSSELL MANUEL, M.D., MSc.

Dr. Manuel is a highly regarded medical doctor with international credentials and licensed in Canada, United Kingdom, Hong Kong, Jamaica, Tanzania, and the United States. He has a degree in public health and has held several key public health positions in Canada. Dr. Manuel also has a Master of Science degree in epidemiology. He has extensive training and experience spanning a number of areas, from public health and research, to preventive medicine programs. Dr. Manuel has practiced medicine and surgery in six countries including Africa, Jamaica, and Hong Kong.

Today, Dr. Manuel is retired from active medical practice after being a researcher and full-time professor of preventive medicine and epidemiology. He occasionally gives guest lectures to medical schools, and is currently a holistic medical consultant to individuals and health professionals. Dr. Manuel has a keen interest in the study of parasites since his Africa days and believes they are a major problem in North America today.

CHAPTER 1

The Parasite Menace

How many people do you know that have some type of chronic health problem? How many of them over the age of 45 are on blood pressure medication, some type of antacid, or something to control their blood sugar? How many people do you know are suffering from chronic fatigue or have some type of cancer? Do you know people who have been seriously ill for months, but doctors can't find anything wrong with them? Do they think it is just stress? With all the money being funneled into research and technology today, it is hard to believe that so many people still have such poor health. Instead of experiencing better health, most of the people living in North America are deteriorating. People may be living longer, but they are not living healthier. There are many factors that contribute to this decline in health, but parasites may be one of the most overlooked causes.

The founding editor of *Prevention Magazine*, J.I. Rodale, once wrote an editorial saying that only those who protect themselves from the steadily increasing burdens of toxic environmental pollution would survive in coming times. In the last century, we have witnessed the progressive poisoning of nature with the chemical by-products of modern life. These chemical changes are not just confined to the areas where they occur. There is evidence of pollution everywhere on Earth, from the largest cities to the remote and isolated South Pole.

Congress has passed a series of laws recently that seriously damages years of valuable health and environmental laws and regulations. More of us will be negatively impacted by environmental hazards that Congress has the power to eliminate. There has been serious dilution of the Clean Water Act, the Clean Air Act, the Safe Drinking Water Act, and the Meat and Poultry Products Inspection Acts. These laws are there to protect the environment and to protect us. One result of all this is the higher incidence of parasitic infection among the American public.

Could It Happen Here?

You probably have never seen a parasite. So, why would you worry about them? Since we have good sanitation, how could we possibly have parasites? The World Health Organization categorizes parasites as among the six most harmful diseases that infect humans. These pathogens now outrank cancer as the number-one killer in the world today and account for much of the illnesses. The magnitude of these infections is absolutely staggering.

You may think that such polluted conditions do not exist in the United States, but you are wrong. Most people think that parasitic infections only occur in distant parts of the world such as impoverished rural areas in third-world countries, or in the tropics. Nothing could be further from the truth. Because of this misconception, many people have overlooked the possibility of parasites as the cause of their illness.

In 1993 hundreds of thousands of people fell ill from the protozoan, *Cryptosporidium,* that infected the city's water system in Milwaukee, Wisconsin. Many people died. In 1994 the Pacific Northwest had an incident of contaminated hamburger meat containing the bacteria *Escherichia coli.* Hundreds of people became ill and two children died. These incidents are happening more often right here in our own country. America needs stronger environmental laws and regulations, not less, or we will not have a healthy future.

Most people recognize the names of parasites such as tapeworms and pinworms, but they are completely unaware of the variety and quantity present in the population as a whole. These potentially harmful parasites, and their effects, are increasing at a rapid rate as the cause of ill health in this country. Parasites should be an important part of every medical evaluation in cases of illness.

What Are Parasites?

Parasites are organisms that live in or on another organism (the host), at the expense of that host, and often compete for nutrition. The host will be injured to some degree from this relationship. The parasites that I refer to in this book are usually the ones that live inside the human body feeding off the food that we provide them, or consuming body tissues and cells. Their sizes range from very small microscopic amebas to very large intestinal worms that can grow to several feet long. Over 100 common types of human parasites are known and a body can host more than one kind at a time. Parasites excrete waste products that may be toxic, and prey on people with weakened immunity. The infection parasites cause usually starts with contaminated water or food, or coming into contact with infected animals or people through fecal-oral contact.

PARASITES CAUSE ILLNESS

The Center for Disease Control and Prevention (CDC) estimates that there are 50 million cases of food-borne illnesses each year and approximately 9,000 people die as a result. Public health officials are not required to report food-related illnesses to the CDC, so we really don't know how many cases there are. Doctors only hear about a few of these cases because many people with food poisoning assume that they have stomach flu and don't go to the doctor for treatment.

Worldwide, parasitic infections that cause diarrhea are the greatest single cause of illness and death. Few people realize the enormous adverse impact of parasites on human well-being. In the United States, diarrhea caused by intestinal parasites is the third leading cause of illnesses. It is hard to believe that parasites can be so prevalent in this country when we have grown up with so may modern sanitary conveniences.

It comes as a surprise to many people when they find out that they have parasites, especially pathogens, living inside them. But this problem is very common and occurs in places and among people who are health-minded. Parasites are no longer a disease of the lower classes. Even the upper middle class in this country are not immune to infection. We have to quit thinking that only the tropical, poor, and unsanitary areas of the world can be infected with parasites.

Parasites have the ability to secrete substances that are toxic to the body. If you have ever experienced acute dysentery caused by these toxins, you know how debilitating the symptoms can be. Toxins give our bodies something else to deal with and increase the process of detoxification. On the other hand, you could have a chronic parasitic infection that secretes such low levels of toxins over a long period that there are not any obvious symptoms produced. Over time, these toxins stress the body and cause a variety of health problems.

Parasites multiply at an incredible rate, with some of them laying thousands of eggs each day. When you consider that many of them can live in a human body for decades, releasing millions of eggs and waste produces over the course of their lifetime, it is hard to believe that parasites don't influence our health in some way.

You might think that if it is so easy to get parasites, why doesn't everyone have them? Well, Most people do have them, whether or not they produce apparent symptoms. You might think that since you seem healthy and not aware of any problems, you could not have parasites. To reach a level of vibrant health, you have to find out if pathogenic parasites are living in you, and then get rid of them.

WHAT DOES A PARASITE EAT?

Not all parasites consume the same diet. Some organisms just love sugar or other simple carbohydrates. If you also love sugar, then it would stand to reason that this is the kind of parasite you would attract. The parasites often eat the nutrients in your body before you get to use them. You are left with what the parasites do not want, the leftovers. They grow healthy and fat, and you starve for nutrition. Parasites can remain in your body, robbing it of nutrients for many years; some have a lifespan of 20 to 30 years. This means that you could have eaten contaminated food 10 years ago and still harbor the same organism somewhere in your digestive tract.

Some parasites get their food from the cells in your body. They attach themselves to these cells and are able to derive their nutrition from the cell itself. These are significantly more dangerous then parasites that stay in the digestive tract, because they can travel to places in the body where they can do damage to vital organs.

HOW LONG CAN A PARASITE LIVE?

You may be shocked to know that parasites can remain in your body for 10, 20, and even 30 years. This has been extensively documented in the medical literature. In one study done in 1979, 600 British former POWs from World War II were examined. Even thirty years later, 15 percent of these soldiers were still infected with a parasite, *Strongyloides*, acquired during that war.

PARASITES WANT TO SURVIVE

Most people are unaware that a parasite lives inside them. This is a good thing, if you are a parasite. After all, it would not be wise for a parasite to let themselves be easily detected. If an organism is going to complete its life cycle, its best interest is served by not being detected. Otherwise, its life would certainly be cut short. All organisms want to live and reproduce, even parasites. They have learned to adapt and mutate when necessary.

COMMON PARASITES

In the United States, the most common human parasites, apart from head lice, are the microscopic protozoa varieties that are transmitted by air, food, water, insects, animals, or other people. One of these tiny virulent parasites, *Giardia lamblia*, found in the waters of lakes, streams, and oceans, is a common cause of traveler's diarrhea. *Entamoeba histolytica* causes dysentery and injury to the liver and lungs. *Blastocystis hominis* is linked to acute and chronic illness, and *Dientamoeba fragilis* is associated with diarrhea, abdominal pains, intense anal itching, and loose stools. Cryptosporidium has become a significant threat to those with low immune function or with AIDS. Then there are the parasitic worms, including pinworms, roundworms, and tapeworms. These are usually acquired from eating contaminated meat.

From just one study conducted in 1995, a West-Coast town found out that even with free worming treatments provided by a Department of Health Clinic, and improved sanitation in most of the homes, there still were many infections from parasites. Despite these community services, whipworm in preschool children increased to 75 percent. The study found that the ameba, *Entamoeba histolytica*, was detected frequently. At five primary schools on the East Coast, 65 percent of the infected children had a roundworm (called whipworm), and 39 percent had more than one parasite. The pathogenic protozoan *Giardia lamblia* was also detected.

WHERE DO PARASITES LIVE?

In a medical book entitled *Animals Parasitic in Man*, by Geoffrey Lapage, originally published in 1957, he comments on how there is no part of the human host that is not visited by some type of para-sitic animal at some time or other during a person's life. No organ is immune. Your blood, your muscles, your heart, your lungs, and your brain are all possible sites for parasitic infestation. About one-third of the parasites in humans live in the digestive tract, and the other two-thirds live somewhere else in the body.

IS THIS PARASITE A PATHOGEN?

Sometimes it is hard to know if a parasite is actually a pathogen or not. Just a few decades ago *Giardia lamblia,* now the leading cause of intestinal parasitic infections in the United States, was not con-sidered a pathogen at all. Now it is. Cryptosporidium was considered a pathogen in animals, now it is also one in humans. Today, *Blastocystis hominis* is often considered a pathogen if the quantities are high enough or the host's immune system is ineffective, but just a couple of years ago it was not considered a pathogen at all. *Blastocystis hominis,* along with some forms of yeast, is often the most frequently found organism in stool samples.

It is thought that there are parasites with different strains, some being pathogens, and some not. Some people harbor organisms such as *Giardia lamblia* or *Entamoeba histolytica,* but do not suffer any apparent symptoms. Other people become very ill even when the organisms detected were not the pathogen strain, such as *Entamoeba coli* or *Endolimax nana.* Could the organism switch from one type to another in order to survive? The health of the host may determine whether or not a particular infection will generate symptoms.

How Do We Get Parasites?

Parasites live everywhere and are commonly transmitted to humans in diverse ways, such as insect bites, walking barefoot, and eating under-cooked meats and fish. Government inspectors do not inspect most of the animals that go to the slaughterhouse. What about salads, or even raw fruits and vegetables? Eating foods raw always increases the risk for parasites. According to the CDC, ill-nesses linked with fruits and vegetables are on the rise. One reason could be the increased demand for fresh produce. We now import 30 billion tons of food a year. Some of the produce comes from devel-oping nations where sanitation facilities are less advanced or they commonly practice the use of human feces as fertilizer (night soil).

The further products travel, the more likely they will pick up illness-causing microbes. It also increases the chance of being contaminated by infected food handlers. Food handlers have been in the news lately because of their role in the spread of parasites. Some people who prepare food, as well as the general population, do not wash their hands after going to the bathroom. When you consider that many of the parasites are spread by fecal-oral contact, this lack of personal hygiene may be one of the greatest factors in the spread of parasites.

Parasites can also get into the body by putting hands in the mouth after being in contact with something that has the parasite in or on it. Sharing drinks, kissing, sexual contact, and even inhaling dust that contains the eggs or cysts of these organisms, are all ways parasites enter the body. It is also possible to get parasites from drinking water from many of the lakes, rivers, streams, and creeks in North America. Close contact with companion pets and other animals is another way to acquire parasites.

How Many People Have Parasites?

Approximately one-half of the population carries at least one form of parasite. Twenty-five percent of these people have an active infection with symptoms. Today, you don't even have to travel to foreign countries to acquire parasites. You can get amebas, giardia, cryptosporidium, pinworms, whipworms, tapeworms and a host of others, without ever getting a passport. Yes, the United States has enjoyed a very high standard of living compared with the rest of the world, yet people living in some parts of this country, especially in the warmer, humid climates, have an infection rate that exceeds the rest of the country.

It is important to understand and be aware of how parasites spread and the sources of potential infection. It makes sense that you will reduce your risk to parasites when you also reduce or eliminate the factors from your environment that promote parasite infection. A healthy immune system is the best protection from catching parasites. Stay healthy by giving your body nourishing foods and supplementing your diet with immune-enhancing vitamins, minerals, and herbs.

Young children are at high risk of getting parasites. Much of their time is spent exploring their world and part of this time is spent by putting their unwashed hands in their mouths. Because of their close relationships with their pets, parasites can be transferred when the cat or dog licks the child with their tongue, after having cleaned themselves first.

TRAVEL BRINGS US CLOSER

Knowing that parasitic infection in the U.S. is a much larger problem than most of us think, we can certainly blame conditions in our own water systems, food processing systems and sanitary conditions. But there are also other factors that have contributed to our current situation concerning parasites. Our world has become a global village now that we can get on a plane and fly to anywhere in the world. Whenever Americans spend time in foreign lands they may become infected with pathogens alien to the United States and bring those pathogens back with them. There is also an increase in immigration of people into the United States; some of these peoples bring parasites that are "native" to their countries. In addition, our lifestyles allow us to eat out, camp in the woods by beautiful streams, put our children in day care centers, have close contact with our pets, and take modern drugs. All of these things put us at a high risk of getting parasites and spreading them all around the world.

Soldiers stationed overseas pick up a variety of parasites and bring them home with them to infect their family and friends. Thousands of troops returning from Southeast Asia and the Arab countries were carrying organisms that made many of them sick. There have been law suits against the Veterans Administration for failing to properly test, diagnose, and treat soldiers for parasitic infections. When more than 500,000 American troops returned from Desert Storm, they were told not to donate blood. This was because they had been exposed to the parasite *Leishmania*, which is spread by sand flies. Hundreds to thousands of Vietnam veterans might still be suffering from undiagnosed parasitic infestation.

It is not unusual for people to acquire their parasites in some far-off country and wait five years or more before their symptoms are identified, and treated, as a parasitic infection. Many parasites go undetected because they don't produce any serious symptoms, or only produce symptoms at one stage in their lives. It is easy to attribute feeling ill to other causes because it can look like a hundred other conditions.

WHAT IS THE RATE OF INFECTION?

It is estimated that Native American reservations have a 50 percent rate of parasitic infections. The elderly anywhere are especially vulnerable. Parasites are an unrecognized cause of much of the malnutrition, fatigue, and diarrhea found in the older population. One study done on low-income immigrants who were acutely ill found 70 percent with parasites. Twenty percent of those infected had disease-producing pathogens.

In a more affluent socioeconomic cross section of chronically ill people, 20 percent tested positive for the presence of parasites. In another study, over one-third of the chronic fatigue syndrome patients tested were found to be infected with *Giardia lamblia*. A link has even been found between HIV and parasites. People with AIDS often have treatment-resistant *Candida albicans* (yeast) due to the impaired immune factors caused by many parasites. A study at the University of Virginia reports that an ameba called *Entamoeba histolytica* produces a substance that attacks the very immune defense cells that can inactivate the HIV virus.

Worldwide, malaria infects 300–600 million people and kills approximately 3 million a year, 1 million a year in Africa alone. The giant intestinal roundworm, *Ascaria,* and the roundworm that causes trichinosis, *Trichinella spiralis,* infect 1 billion each. Six hundred million people are estimated to be infected with either *Schistosoma,* a blood fluke, or *Filariasis,* a worm infection of the blood or lymphatic system. Some authorities estimate that 55 million children in the United States have some type of worms.

What Will Your Doctor Do?

It is usually a shock to any person when they see worms being passed in their stool. Sometimes all that is seen are parts of worms, not the whole intact body. But not all parasites can be seen without the aid of a microscope. When you rush to your physician with the news that you saw something strange in the toilet after having a bowel movement, you will probably be talking to someone who received very little or no training in diagnosing and treating parasitic infections. If you go to your physician with symptoms of diarrhea or fever, you will most likely receive medication to just stop the symptoms, without ever finding the real cause.

How can any real cure be possible when the parasite is still there?

For many weeks, months, or even years you continue to have symptoms. You will probably be subjected to many unnecessary laboratory tests, and possibly be hospitalized, and even have surgery suggested, because your doctor is baffled as to what is causing your illness. No one thought it could be some type of protozoa or worm causing your diarrhea or fever.

Even if your doctor thinks that you have parasites, it is likely that the results of testing will be negative. What does this mean? For one thing, the stool sample is usually sent to a local lab that does not specialize in the detection of parasites. At the present time many medical testing procedures for most parasites are only positive 20 percent of the time. Sometimes this is due to poor laboratory technique, not enough different stool samples, using the wrong test, or not catching the parasite in a phase that is easily detected. There are not even tests for all the parasites that can live in your body, so you probably have more parasites present then any test will confirm. Of over 1,000 species of parasites that could infect humans, only about 40 to 50 have tests available to detect them. Since there are specialty parasite laboratories that do use more sophisticated and accurate detection methods, it is important that doctors know about them if they hope to get a correct diagnosis.

But what if you did find out which parasites were present? Would your doctor know which medication to take or how much and how often? Usually, there are only a few physicians that know anything about these organisms, and they only treat the problem with pharmaceutical drugs. Antiparasitic drugs often will not kill more than one or two different types of parasites, and tend to have toxic side effects. If you are infected with several different types of parasites, it may be too harmful to kill all of them at the same time. Many parasites can be treated with less toxic, yet effective, alternatives.

If you do not take the correct medication in the correct dosage, you might only cause the parasite to move from one organ of the body to another. To survive, some parasites will just move to another location that is not exposed to the medication. In the case of tapeworms, if you do not use a therapy that removes the entire tapeworm from the small intestine and the head remains, the entire worm will grow back.

Symptoms of Parasitic Infection

Part of detecting the presence of a parasite in the body is being able to read the body's signals and know how to interpret them. Maybe you have not been paying enough attention to your symptoms or you think that something else is causing the problem. It is amazing that so many people think that having chronic digestive problems, gas, constipation, skin rashes, pains in the stomach area, fatigue, and other "vague" symptoms are just something you have to live with. These symptoms can come from anywhere in the body because parasites can occur anywhere. No organ or tissue is immune from their infestation or from their toxic waste products.

Parasitic infections contribute to a variety of major diseases, including Crohn's disease, ulcerative colitis, arthritis, rheumatoid symptoms, chronic fatigue syndrome, and AIDS. A number of digestive complaints such as diarrhea and irritable bowel syndrome, are linked to past or present parasitic infections. It could look like food or environmental allergies that develop for no apparent reason.

In one study, 50 percent of the people suffering from irritable bowel syndrome had intestinal parasites. The majority of them were considered "cured" when the parasite was treated. This percentage is even higher for people with chronic fatigue syndrome. Any person with chronic gastrointestinal complaints such as bloating, diarrhea, abdominal pain, excessive gas, chronic constipation, multiple allergies especially to food, and unexplained fatigue, should be screened for intestinal parasites.

CAN I BE REINFECTED?

The really distressing thing about parasites is that you can get rid of them, or most of them, but you can easily be reinfected. Married couples tend to have the same ones. When one person is treated for the parasitic infection, they are often reinfected by their spouse. It is extremely important that both be treated at the same time. In many cases, the children should be treated along with their parents.

CAN PARASITES CAUSE CANCER?

Dr. Hulda Clark, Ph.D., N.D., who has doctorate degrees in physiology and naturopathic medicine, says that parasites can cause significant disorders, not just mere signs or symptoms of their presence. This researcher has made the startling statement that parasites can be the cause of cancer. She also states in her trilogy of books that parasites and pollution are the sources of all illnesses. In *The Cure for All Diseases,* she writes that even a person with a long list of symptoms, from chronic fatigue to mental problems, could be suffering from only two direct causes: they have in them pollutants and/or parasites. She also says that it is the human intestinal fluke that is causing cancer. If you kill this parasite, the cancer stops immediately and the tissue becomes normal again.

Why Do We Neglect the Parasite Problem ?

In spite of some efforts to control parasites, their global impact has not been appreciably reduced for a variety of reasons. In addition, immigrants and people with depressed immune systems are showing an increase in protozoa and infections with worms. Why are parasitic infections among the world's greatest neglected diseases? The illusion is that it can't be happening because no one is really talking about it. You don't hear the newspapers and television stations reporting it enough. You don't see people asking for donations to research parasites. When a topic is rarely discussed, who is going to take it seriously?

There is little research being done to stop the spread of parasitic infection. Funding is very low for any research into this area, even if parasites are the single most undiagnosed health challenge in the history of the human race. We have a tremendous parasite problem right here in the United Sates, even if it is not being addressed. Because of the increase in pollution and environmental poisons, parasites of all kinds are invading our bodies. It takes constant vigilance and a change in lifestyle if you want to remain free from them.

CHAPTER 2

Do I Have Parasites?

Some people call parasites the "great masquerader." Many types are so well adapted to living in their human host that no obvious symptoms are presented. Since many of the symptoms of parasite infection are nonspecific and resemble so many other conditions, it is very easy to misdiagnosed the cause of illness. If your health problems persist, think parasites!

When you last saw you physician for an illness, did anyone ask you what you ate or if you had a preference for rare steak? Did they ask you about your recent travel plans to other countries? Did anyone even hint that the real cause of your health concerns might be related to parasites? At a professional medical meeting, one expert told an audience that worms, and other parasites, are the unsuspected cause of many illnesses.

According to the American Medical Association, physicians only correctly diagnose a disease 16 percent of the time; that's one out of six. The average medical laboratory is lucky to diagnose parasites 20 percent of the time. It there any wonder a physician might not connect symptoms, especially vague ones, to parasites?

The idea of parasites being the cause of so many illnesses is not receiving its deserved attention. There are only a few facilities that specialize in parasitology. Recent outbreaks of bacteria (*Entamoeba coli*) and viruses (bird flu in Hong Kong and ebola in Africa) will only expedite the development of better organism detection.

The longer the parasite is in the human body, the more likely there will be some damage, depending on the target site of infection. If the parasite is in the intestinal tract, one of the things that the body will do is to produce more mucus to protect the intestinal cells. Unfortunately, this coating interferes with digestion, leading to the malabsorption of important nutrients, particularly fats and fat-soluble vitamins such as vitamins A and E. As the parasites continue to flourish, they take more nutrition and leave us malnourished. The more severe the infestation, the more severe the deficiencies. You are not only feeding a parasite within you, you are also absorbing the toxic waste products it produces. The waste material from just one tapeworm can make someone feel ill. Some authorities think that the waste products from flukes contribute to the formation of cancer.

The most commonly reported symptoms of parasite infection are diarrhea and abdominal pain. Specific symptoms are frequently associated with certain organisms such as fever with malaria, but almost any symptom can manifest with almost any parasite. There are many cases in the literature associating parasites with allergies. Sometimes it is hard to tell if the parasite causes the allergy or a person with many allergies is more at risk of getting parasites.

The following are examples of the symptoms people have after contracting parasites. These only illustrate how easily and innocently we may become infected.

- Hundreds of veterans returning from the Persian Gulf came back with puzzling symptoms, including fatigue, joint pain, hair loss, a rash, bleeding gums and liver problems. The prime suspect was a treatable parasitic infection from sand fly bites called leishmaniasis.
- A young boy picked up a worm infestation from his pets by sleeping with them. He suffered from constant fatigue, bloating, and irritability. One specialist suggested he had leukemia. When the animals were kept out of his bed and an intestinal cleansing and treatment for parasites was done, the boy quickly recovered and was a happy child again in a couple of weeks.
- A woman with a recurring breast infection improved after getting rid of a roundworm infestation.
- A teenager suffered from wheezing, coughing, chronic crying and depression, and an allergy to many foods, as well as dust and mold. He lived in close contact with two small dogs; both had worms. After he and the dogs were treated, the problems decreased quickly.
- A woman diagnosed with myasthenia gravis (a condition marked

by muscular weakness and progressive fatigue) improved dramatically after passing a large tapeworm.

- One 7-year-old boy began having abdominal pain on the left side,
with episodes lasting from 20 minutes to an hour. He had a severe
attack at school that lasted for several hours. After being taken to
a physician, nothing was found during a physical exam except
some tenderness in the abdominal area. The laboratory tests all
came back negative. Everyone thought that the boy was just faking
his symptoms to get out of going to school. When the symptoms
didn't let up, he was tested by a facility that specializes in parasites.
Large amounts of *Dientamoeba fragilis* were found. One of the main
symptoms that this organism causes is abdominal pain. After the
child was treated, there were not any further symptoms.

- A family was traveling through California where they stopped at a
roadside stand to buy some fresh peaches. They ate the peaches
without washing them first. By the next day they all had diarrhea
and abdominal pain. When they returned home a few days later,
they all visited their physician and lab tests did not reveal the
cause of their suffering. Then they were tested by a specialty lab
that tested for parasites. Three were found: *Blastocystis hominus,*
Entamoeba histolytica, and *Ascaris lumbricoides.* After these parasites
were treated, the entire family were free of any symptoms.

- A woman went to Mexico and acquired a protozoa infection during the trip. By the time she returned to the United States, she
had a fever and was violently ill. She was very dehydrated and
began to have seizures. This was all because of a parasitic infection. It took a couple of months to resolve all of her symptoms.

In the absence of symptoms and a positive laboratory test, it can
be difficult to diagnose the presence of parasites. It is common that
over half of the people with parasites are without obvious symptoms,
but there still may be some nonspecific ones that could suggest that
parasites are somewhere in the body:

- Foul-smelling stools that are worse in the afternoon and evening.
- Bowel habits have changes over several days or weeks or even
months. Now there are soft or watery bowel movements or occasional constipation.
- The presence of abdominal cramps and rumblings and gurglings
in the stomach area at times different from hunger and eating.

- Pains in the chest or heartburn that weren't there before.
- Sore and swollen breast not related to the menstrual cycle.
- Flulike symptoms, such as coughing wheezing and fever.
- Food allergies to many different types of foods.
- Itching around the anus, especially at night.
- Losing weight, yet have a ravenous appetite.

The following are some additional signs and symptoms of parasitic infections:

- anemia
- asthma
- autoimmune disease
- bedwetting
- bloating
- blood in stools
- chronic fatigue
- Crohn's disease
- depression
- digestive problems
- dysentery
- excessive nose picking
- feeling full in the stomach
- flatulence
- grinding teeth at night
- headaches
- hungry feeling all the time
- immune dysfunction
- impaired thinking
- inflammatory bowel disease
- intestinal obstruction
- irritable bowel disease
- itchy skin, ears, nose, anus
- joint/muscle aches and pains
- loss of appetite
- low-back pain
- nausea
- nervousness
- rash, itching of skin
- restlessness even in sleep
- shortness of breath
- sleeping disturbances
- sore mouth and gums
- stomach aches or burns
- toxic feeling
- vomiting

CHAPTER 3

What Puts Us At Risk?

There are unsuspected risks of parasite infections in and around the home. Some are easily identifiable, while others may be more difficult to detect. The follow sections examine several areas of possible sources of parasite infection.

ANIMALS

If there are raccoons in your area, they may be infected with roundworms. Many wild animals, including squirrels and possums, also carry parasites. Small children tend to handle and chew on objects that may be contaminated with these animals' feces. Children should not eat dirt or be allowed to play in yards, playgrounds, or sandboxes where animals roam and defecate. Certainly, don't walk barefoot in these areas, especially in warm, moist and sandy soil. Wear gloves when gardening, because the soil can be contaminated with the eggs or cysts of parasites.

Pets have a unique relationship with us. They share our homes, eat off our plates, get on our furniture and kitchen counters, and sleep in our beds. It is not surprising that we can get parasites from them. Don't let your children kiss, or be kissed or licked by their pets. This goes for adults, too. Keep your children, especially infants and toddlers, away from pets that have not been dewormed regularly. Don't sleep near pets if they have not been dewormed. Sometimes, we are just careless when cleaning up after them. Unless you wash your hands after every contact with your pet, you are putting yourself at risk for infection. See the chapter "Animal Care" for more information.

ANTIBIOTICS

Taking antibiotics disturbs the balance of intestinal microflora and makes the host more susceptible to parasites. The excessive use of antibiotics also encourages the spread of parasites by lowering the body's own ability to fight back. This makes it hard to develop a strong and healthy immune system. Using antibiotics in livestock has compounded the problems by creating antibiotic-resistant organisms in the food we eat.

FOOD HANDLERS

The risk of parasitic infections from our food is growing rapidly. Today, people eat more exotic foods, travel abroad, and frequent restaurants that employ immigrants from other countries such as Asia, Central and South America, the Caribbean, Vietnam, and Haiti, where the parasite rate of infection is very high. Many people come to this country unskilled and end up working for minimum wage in kitchens preparing foods or picking food crops in the fields. It is common for illegal immigrants to find jobs for low wages somewhere in the food industry.

They also find themselves in a foreign country with an unfamiliar language and may not be able to read signs telling them to wash their hands before handling food items or after using the bathroom. Infected food handlers, especially untrained or careless restaurant employees, do pass along their parasites. So beware! If restaurant eating is part of your lifestyle, you probably have been exposed to parasites.

Immigrants also find work as babysitters or housekeepers, or as a nanny in the home. This was the case of a worker from South American who came from a region where pork tapeworms were common. She brought the parasites with her to New York causing a mysteriously illness in the family members she was working for. Pork tapeworms were forming cysts in the brains of her employers, causing seizures. The housekeeper had contaminated the food she prepared with tapeworm eggs and infected the entire family. Screen all employees in your home, such as the nanny, maid or housekeeper for parasites. This is particularly important if this person is preparing food for you and your family.

When the contamination of food occurs at the retail level, it usually involves improper handling. Grocery stores sometimes put lettuce in a tub of water to make them look better, but one bad head in the tub can contaminate the rest of the lettuce. It is not unusual to see stores place herbs, such as cilantro, into a container filled with water to keep them fresh. The water used is usually unfiltered tap water.

Are people who handle your food wearing gloves? Have you noticed that many of the same people who serve you in restaurants, grocery stores, and other places where you buy your food, also handle your money? This lack of sanitation increases your exposure rate to infectious diseases such as parasites. All food handlers, whether it be in restaurants, cafeterias, schools, hospitals, or other institutions, need to be examined for parasites. Anyone handling food should be tested.

HYGIENE PRACTICES

The following hygiene practices frequently influence the extent of invasion by parasites:

- Always wash your hands, top and bottom, with soap and water prior to eating or handling food, and after going to the bathroom. It is also important to wash your hands after changing a child's diaper. Get in the habit of not putting your hands in your mouth unless you wash them first. The best hygiene practice is not to put your hands in your mouth at anytime.
- Do not brush your teeth with the local tap water and keep your toothbrush away from contaminated areas. It is best to keep it in a sealed container in a cabinet. Always keep the cap on the toothpaste.
- Have your children wash their hands after playing outside. Teach them not to put their hands or toys in their mouths. Clean toys regularly with mild, soapy water.
- Teach your children to always wash their hands in soapy water after contact with household pets. It is best to keep your children away from pets until they are dewormed.
- Wash your hands after handling raw animal flesh, including meat, fish, and crustaceans including shrimp. Use bleach or a disinfectant to clean surfaces. Always wash your hands after touching any food. Even fruits and vegetables come from parts of the world where they can be contaminated by food handlers or by the practice of using human fertilizer.
- Use a separate cutting board for preparing meat and vegetables.

Use one that can be either disinfected or put in the dishwasher. Wash utensils thoroughly after cutting meat or fish, but don't place them on the kitchen counter while cooking and preparing food. Place the utensils on something, such as a ceramic holder, that can be disinfected.

- Keep children's fingernails short and clean. Keep a nail brush by the sink especially if your work around children, food, or the elderly. Teach your children to use a nail brush, too.
- Wipe off the toilet seat before sitting on it or use paper liners or toilet paper between you and the toilet seat. If you are not able to do this, then squat over the toilet seat without touching it. Don't forget the potty for children. Pinworm eggs can be found even under the toilet seat, so do not touch the seat with your hands. Remember to disinfect under the seat when cleaning. Scrub the toilet seat daily that any infected person uses.
- Be cautious around saunas, hot tubs, and water baths. Don't sit bare-bottom in the warm water on the edges because parasites can live there.
- Never use non-sterilized water to clean contact lenses. It is best to use sterilized preparations for all cleansing and disinfecting purposes. Don't wear contact lenses when swimming if possible.
- If your child already has parasites such as pinworms, it is important to do additional hygiene practices because this parasite is easy to spread to others. Be sure they bathe daily, don't let them share towels, use a different towel for the face then for the rest of the body, wear close-fitting underwear at all times even under pajamas, and do not let them sleep in a bed with others. The bed clothing needs to be washed daily.
- Clean and vacuum daily to remove eggs from the floors and carpets.
- Keep all rooms well ventilated, especially the bedroom of the infected person.
- If you can, superheat the house for a day to 95° F to kill the egg embryos. It is best to leave the house during this time (be sure all pets are out of the house as well). If you can't superheat the whole house, you can at least heat the infected person's room.

JOB-RELATED CAUSES

- Some jobs lend themselves to putting a person at a higher risk of parasitic infections. These include electricians, plumbers, and other workers who crawl beneath raised buildings where animals have left their feces.

- People who are employed overseas, as well as family members who accompany them, should be examined for parasites. At least twice a year get a complete blood count, liver function tests, and be examined for parasites. People who return to this country after working overseas can harbor parasites and infect the whole family.
- Anyone working in and around animals should get examined for parasites regularly. This would include people working in animal kennels, pet shops, zoos, veterinary clinics, and cattle feed lots. It should also include gardeners and sanitation workers, as well as animal trainers.
- Day-care workers should be checked regularly for parasites. It is especially important to maintain good hygiene practices when changing diapers, and then handling food or toys. All employees should routinely wash their hands and scrub under the fingernails after using the bathroom and changing diapers. Teach children to have good hygiene practices as well. Clean toys and water faucets daily. Change diapers only in one area to reduce the chance of contamination. Disinfect this area after each changing with a soapy water solution. Keep children at home who have symptoms of diarrhea.
- Food handlers in restaurants, hotels, and school or workplace cafeterias should be required to undergo parasite testing.

LIFESTYLE

When a person eats a poor diet, it increases susceptibility to parasites. A sluggish bowel encourages imbalances in the intestine's microflora and this encourages the overgrowth of pathogens. Chronic stress and fatigue weakens the human body. If you eat out a lot or have pets, it is important to have a complete parasite examination at least twice a year. See the chapter "Diet and Digestion" for more information.

RECREATION

Parasites are found in recreational waters, lakes, and streams, as well as swimming pools. With the rising popularity of water sports, infected human waste in the water has become a growing problem. It is easy for swimmers to swallow a mouthful of water. That water may contain parasites from the local livestock that defecated into the water upstream. What about the person that washed off an infected soiled diaper in the lake you are swimming in? Drinking "raw" water is an open invitation to parasites.

Some parasites thrive in the cold rushing mountain streams and beautiful lakes that dot this country. When you last went camping, did you wash off your dishes or perhaps some food in the tranquil lake next to where you were staying? Parasite cysts are very tough and can survive easily in cold water. Other parasites love the sun. Sunbathers who recline on wet sand, and children who like to play on the wet, sandy beach are easy prey for hookworm larvae if the area has become contaminated.

SEXUAL PRACTICES

Studies are now looking at the relationship between acquiring parasites and AIDS. The AIDS virus is probably not causing the disease all by itself. Other factors may make it more likely that exposure to the virus will also create an environment that will develop into AIDS. Some researchers indicate that it is the continuing spread of parasites among homosexual men that is a major contributor to the spread of AIDS. This theory has important practical value, because it suggests ways to reduce the risk and spread of AIDS.

Check with your local health department or through various organizations concerned with AIDS, or other sexually transmitted diseases, to see if they have an active program for the eradication of parasites. Some pharmaceutical drugs used to treat parasites can cause serious side effects, especially in cases where the person who has parasites also has AIDS. These medications must be monitored carefully. It is best to consult a physician who has experience treating parasites.

The main difference between people who become HIV positive, and those who don't, is whether or not they had a suppressed immune system to start with. In people with good immunity the virus does not develop far enough to be life threatening. Parasites have the ability to suppress the immune system, maybe as one way to protect themselves against a hostile environment. Parasites can activate the white blood cells, called helper T-cells, into attacking healthy tissues of the body for long periods of time. Laboratory studies have found that the AIDS virus becomes more likely to infect a person when these cells are activated. Minor diseases and infections do not usually activate the T-cells for very long, only a few days.

After parasites damage the intestinal tract, it may allow the AIDS virus to get into the bloodstream easier. This damage to the intestinal wall called "leaky gut syndrome" allows undigested proteins in food to get into the bloodstream, causing allergies and further activating the T-cells. With the parasites causing intestinal damage there is the likely chance of malabsorption, resulting in malnutrition. This weakens the body and the immune system.

It is important to test any sexual partner(s) for parasites. Both need to get treated at the same time to prevent reinfection. The safe-sex guidelines for preventing AIDS will not always stop transmission of parasites. Handling condoms after use is just one way to transmit parasites. Even small amounts of feces, too small to be seen or smelled, can contaminate hands or other parts of the body, or other objects. It then gets into the mouth during eating, smoking, or other activities, causing the spread of the parasites.

The *New England Journal of Medicine* drew a connection between AIDS and epidemic outbreaks of amebas two years prior to the San Francisco AIDS outbreak. Other researchers pointed out that amebas produce a substance that ruptures immune defense cells that normally engulf the HIV virus. Once these cells rupture, the virus spreads throughout the system. Since the incidence of many other parasites has also increased, this could be fatal in a person with AIDS.

Even if parasites have nothing to do with the direct cause of AIDS, it is still important to diagnose and treat any organisms that could be in the body causing malnutrition and immune deficiency. Many physicians tend to not treat an individual if only nonpathogenic organisms are found. Maybe, this is the wrong thing to do. Sometimes, nonpathogenic organisms in sufficient numbers or in certain strains can and do cause pathology. No matter what treatment you use, it is important to follow-up with additional tests to see if the treatment really worked.

Even in relationships where there is little chance of contact with the AIDS virus, it is important to be tested periodically to see if parasites are present. Just due to different types of sexual practices, it is possible to acquire parasites and pass them on to a sexual partner. Prevention of sexually transmitted parasitic disease depends on practicing safe sex and avoiding certain sexual practices.

Today, it is common practice to have many sexual partners and to conduct a variety of sexual practices that greatly increase the risk of parasites. The prevalence of anal/oral sex has opened the door to the spread of parasitic infection. Sex toys may contain contaminated fecal matter. The life cycle of many parasites depends on this practice by spreading to the hands, mouth, and body through fecal contamination.

Some basic hygiene practices can prevent the passing of parasites. Carefully wash hands after bowel movements. Clean the anal region before and after sex. Any sexual activity that brings a person in contact with the feces of an infected partner greatly increases the risk for parasites. Individuals who practice oral sex need to use a latex barrier (dental dam or condom cut lengthwise) or should avoid oral sex altogether. Regardless of sexual preference, always wear a condom when engaging in sexual intercourse.

WOMEN: SPECIFIC CAUSES

Women need to take special preventive measures because of their unique anatomical design. Have your doctor check for cervical pinworms and roundworms during your yearly pap smear. This is especially important if you have frequent sexual partners. Always wipe from front to back after urinating. Get tested for *Toxoplasma gondii*, which causes toxoplasmosis if you are pregnant or planning to get pregnant. It is important not to be exposed to cats or soiled kitty pans. In addition, have someone else clean the kitty pan and have your cat checked for *Toxoplasma gondii.*

WORLD TRAVEL

World travel has increased and many people are traveling to areas where they come into contact with contaminated food and water. As people from other regions of the world, especially from the South Pacific, Mexico, South America, Asia, and Haiti, along with foreign students, diplomats, immigrants, and returning soldiers, come to this country, guess what they bring with them? Someone doesn't have to have symptoms to be a carrier of these diseases. People without symptoms can be just as infectious, and sometimes even more, than those people with full-blown symptoms.

Don't drink the water or use ice made from unfiltered water. This is good advice no matter where you travel. Even municipal water treatment plants in this country are often inadequate and harbor pathogens such as cryptosporidium. Look at what happened in Milwaukee, Wisconsin, a few years ago. Over 300,000 people became infected with this parasite and some became severely ill, and a few even died. Take along a portable water filter or drink only from reliable bottled water sources. Avoid ice cubes in your drinks unless they are made from bottled or filtered water. Do not brush your teeth with the local tap water. Eat only cooked or peeled fruits and vegetables.

Avoid wearing any kind of scent when traveling, especially in the tropics of Africa, Asia, or the Middle East. This includes deodorants that smell, hair sprays, perfumes, aftershave, etc. Keep the skin covered, especially at night. The mosquitoes that carry malaria are found only between dusk and dawn. Sleep under well-screened netting.

International travel is always a potential source for parasitic infection. You may not realize that you can return with an insidious infection like malaria, roundworm, or blood flukes. Over half of the people reported with symptoms of parasitic infections had some foreign travel within the last 5 years. Here are some examples of where people traveled and what parasite they acquired:

- People who were infected with at least two parasites including *Blastocystis hominis* and *Entamoeba sp.* had most frequently traveled to Mexico, Europe, East Asia, and Central and South America.
- Among people who were only infected with *Blastocystis hominis,* most of them had traveled to the Indian subcontinent including Nepal. Some travelers visited more than just one country during their travels including Mexico, East Asia (Thailand and Indonesia), Central and South America, the Caribbean, Canada, Hawaii, the Middle East, and Australia.
- People traveling to Nepal returned with such severe cases of *Blastocystis hominis* infections that they had not resolved even after 2 years of treatment. A study in Katmandu, Nepal, implicates *Blastocystis hominis* as the cause of 56 out of 189 people who had traveler's diarrhea.
- *Cyclospora cayetanensis* infected people who traveled mostly to Europe, Mexico, Thailand, Nepal, Haiti, and Peru.
- *Entamoeba coli* infected people who traveled most frequently to Mexico, Europe and the Caribbean, as well as Central and South America.
- *Entamoeba hartmanni* infected people who traveled most frequently to Mexico and Europe. The distribution of *Entamoeba hartmanni* is limited, but there are reports of up to a 35 percent prevalence in Mexico City.

- *Entamoeba histolytica* infected people traveling most frequently to Mexico and Europe and somewhat less frequently to East Asia and the Caribbean. People concurrently infected with *Entmoeba histolytica/Entmoeba dispar* and *Entamoeba spp.* traveled most frequently to Mexico, Europe, and the Indian subcontinent. Central and South America are recognized endemic areas of *Entamoeba histolytica*. Travelers to and immigrants from these areas are at a particularly high risk.

Before you go on a trip it is important to plan. Contact the Center for Disease Control in Atlanta, Georgia, (404) 629-3311, and their Traveler's Health Section to obtain guides to regional diseases in the areas where you will be traveling. If you travel frequently, eat out a lot, or hike or backpack into the woods, have a complete parasite examination at least twice a year.

CHAPTER 4

Diet and Digestion

Our diet and nutritional status may be of major importance in determining the outcome of a parasitic infection. The real tragedy is that the majority of people living in the United States, one of the most affluent countries in the world, fail to meet even federal standards for a healthy, balanced diet. Just one percent meet all the recommendations, only 36 percent consumed the recommended 3-5 servings of vegetables each day, and only 26 percent regularly eat 2-4 servings of fruit daily.

The amounts of processed sugars added to the diet is quickly increasing. Many parasites, including roundworms, thrive on a body that is constipated and eating sweet foods, even natural sources such as juice. Diets high in other refined carbohydrates and other processed foods, as well as pesticides, additives and dyes, encourage an environment for parasites. This type of lifestyle usually includes other pollutants that weaken the body. It is no wonder that the immune system is failing to defend itself agains parasites.

Today, the lifestyle of the average person keeps the body chemistry out of balance. The pathways become exhausted and undigested food can get into the bloodstream. The immune system looks at this undigested food as a foreign invader, comes to our defense, and escorts this intruder out of the body. Our body is not designed to handle this type of stress on a daily basis. It puts excessive demands on the immune system and makes us more prone to parasitic infections, as well as other health problems. It also congests the lymphatic system and decreases its ability to carry off toxins from the body.

A well-balance diet improves immune function and can defend the body against parasites. This means a diet high in natural fiber including plenty of vegetables and fruits, but low in fat, sugar, and refined carbohydrates. It is very important to maintain a moderate amount of complete protein and unrefined complex carbohydrates. This would include beans, starchy root vegetables, and a variety of whole grains and nuts. The diet should also contain green leafy vegetables with low amounts of meat and dairy. Include antiparasitic foods such as garlic and pumpkin seeds.

It is also important to get adequate amounts of water and essential fatty acids in the form of safflower, sunflower, and flax oil. Raw goat's milk may be effective in the treatment of parasites because it contains the immune factors called secretory IgA and IgG antibodies. Avoid foods that are known to cause reactions. It is always best to exclude anything with alcohol, sugar or caffeine.

Some parasites seem to occur less when there is adequate dietary fiber in the diet, especially insoluble fiber. Infected animals placed on a high fiber diet, even for 24 hours, were able to decrease their population of parasites in the intestines. Fiber keeps some of the parasites from attaching to the intestinal wall or moves them out of the intestinal tract to be eliminated with the feces. This reduces their ability to establish and sustain colonies. Fiber also keeps the bowels healthy and can positively affect the growth of beneficial bowel flora, giving the parasites some competition.

When your diet includes adequate fiber and water, it leads to a bowel transit time that eliminates waste properly from the intestinal tract. This leads to a healthy gut lining so that you are less prone to allergies. This ensures fewer toxins in the digestive tract and the liver. Keeping the bowel environment healthy is one of the best ways to eradicate parasites. When a person is healthy, they can weather many more challenges, as well as prevent disease from developing.

When people hear the term "balanced diet," they usually think of eating foods belonging to all of the basic food groups. There is another aspect of balance in the diet that is essential to health. This balance has to do with the acid and alkaline levels in the foods we eat. If the foods we put into our bodies are too acidic or too alkaline, they are not properly assimilated. The typical American diet is usually highly acidic. This explains the success of antacid tablets, since they are alkaline and neutralize acidic conditions. This may bring temporary relief, but the stomach needs acid in order to digest the food. The practice of neutralizing stomach acid with pills results in more digestion problems and creates a great environment for parasites. For additional information on acid-alkaline balance, see my book, *Allergies and Holistic Treatments*.

Maintaining a proper acid-alkaline balance is essential for a healthy life and vitality, and is probably one of the most important things you can do with your diet. A proper balance is normally maintained through the body's buffering system. This ability depends on a healthy digestive system, as well as a healthy liver. Poor assimilation and elimination, lack of hydrochloric acid and other digestive enzymes, severe infection or illness, heavy smoking, drinking alcohol, or drug consumption, all interfere with this buffering system. When the body becomes either too acidic or too alkaline, its mineral relationship becomes upset, and may express itself with symptoms. Some of the non-food causes of an acid system are parasites, allergies, high stress, a toxic environment, a sedentary lifestyle, illness, or a combination of several different stressors on the body at the same time.

A healthy body keeps large alkaline reserves to meet emergency demands. A body can function normally and sustain health only in the presence of these adequate alkaline reserves and the proper acid-alkaline ratio in all the body tissues and the blood. Eating the wrong type of foods depletes these reserves. The best ratio of alkaline to acid foods for the body is approximately 4 to 1; four parts alkaline foods to one part acid foods. With such an ideal ratio, the body has a strong resistance to disease and parasites. A person with an acid body chemistry recovers quicker from illness if they begin to eat more alkaline foods.

Figs are very alkaline, as are most fruits, green leafy vegetables, root vegetables, herbs, and spices. The following common foods are also more alkaline that they are acidic. Included in this list are molasses, olives, soybeans, cucumbers, spinach, real maple syrup, beets, avocados, almonds, carrot, chestnuts, potatos, cantaloupe, various types of lettuce, pineapples, coconut, baked beans, cabbage, cherries, and others. Sprouted seeds and grains become more alkaline in the process of sprouting. Just because a fruit has an acid taste does not indicate that its reaction in the body is acidic. It may breakdown to being alkaline. Honey and raw sugars are also alkaline, but in excessive amounts and high concentrations they become acid formers.

Now, on the acid side of food, egg yolk is one of the most acid-forming foods. Most grains are acid-forming, except millet and buckwheat. Most carbohydrates, including noodles, are also acid forming. Some of the most acidic foods are wheat germ, chicken, eggs, beef, liver, lamb chops, cod fish, coffee, and most forms of processed sugar. Other acid forming foods are alcohol, cola drinks, catsup, cocoa, flour products, mustard, and pasta. Dairy products are fairly acidic, including all cheeses, ice cream, custards, and pasteurized or homogenized milk. Some fruits are acid forming including prunes, cranberries, and plums, and the juice made from fruit. All foods with added sugars become acidic. Alcohol, drugs, aspirin, and tobacco are also acid-forming. White or acetic vinegar is very acid whereas balsamic vinegar is low acid and rice vinegar is the lowest in acidic properties. The coffee with the lowest degree of acidity is Kona coffee, but most coffees are still acidic.

People with chronic disease and symptoms almost always have an unhealthy diet. There may be other factors related to why they are sick, but a poor diet will certainly not provide a body with the nutrition it needs to heal itself. A poor diet leads to a sluggish bowel system that results in unhealthy bowel flora with an increase in gut permeability, leading to more yeast and parasites finding a good home. The combination of all of these factors causes a tremendous overload of toxins in the body. When parasites secrete their toxins into an already overloaded system, you are going to feel sick and take longer to heal.

Our lifestyles are changing. More and more people are eating out. Because of the fondness for eating fish, beef, and pork raw or undercooked in dishes called sushi, steak tartar, and cerviche, the risk of tapeworm infection is increasing. Salad bars are popular in many restaurants. This puts us at a high risk of being exposed to microbes that are normally killed when cooked. It might be better to skip the salad bars all together, and only order well-cooked foods.

It is important to use caution when using water from mountains, streams, or creeks, because of the possibility of contamination with parasites. Do not buy bottled, canned, or even fresh fruits or vegetables, or other food products, that have been washed in questionable water. This includes all fruits and vegetables imported from countries where parasites are commonly found. Any food that has been washed with water contaminated with parasitic cysts can also become contaminated.

Especially when traveling abroad or into mountainous regions of the United States, you may want to take along a portable water filter, or only drink from reliable bottled water sources. Eat only cooked or peeled fruits and vegetables. Avoid ice cubes made from unfiltered water. They are usually made from the local tap water and can contain parasites. Avoid regional foods and special dishes that include raw, pickled, smoked, or dried fish, crabs, and crayfish. Cook all meats thoroughly. Microwave cooking frequently undercooks fish and other meats, allowing the larvae to survive and enter the human intestinal system.

A healthy digestive tract certainly influences whether or not parasites have a good environment in which to flourish. If you could spread out the digestive tract, you would be amazed at how large the surface is; about the size of a football field. It is the place where the body interfaces with the environment. This explains why any event that occurs in the digestive tract has such an immense effect upon the entire body. Infections to parasites are more likely if a person has poor digestive system function.

The digestive and intestinal tract system is a complex and dynamic ecosystem where the beneficial bowel flora is a major component. Beneficial, and not so beneficial, organisms are influenced by many factors: the interaction between the different bowel flora, exposure to foreign substances, foods provided, composition and amount of digestive enzymes, mucus production, and status of the intestinal lining. Changes in these factors and the nutritional status of the host will affect this environment. When the digestive tract is working properly, the digestive enzymes will help to destroy the parasites.

Most parasites enter the body through the stomach so having a healthy amount of stomach acid is important. Few pathogenic microorganisms can survive this digestive enzyme, but many factors contribute to a lack of it. Some of the factors contributing to low levels of stomach acid are overgrowths of the yeast, *Candida albicans,* heavy metal toxins such as lead, taking antacids, stress, and some bacteria that can live in the stomach causing it not to produce stomach acid. Americans are particularly vulnerable to parasites because so many people suffer from stomach function problems.

Someone who has a low acid level in the stomach not only can't digest their food properly, but can't kill the parasites coming through. That's what the hydrochloric acid does. It sterilizes the food and kills off all the germs. If it is not effective at doing just that, the parasites can pass along into the intestines. That's one reason why children are prone to parasites. Their digestive system is not as mature as adults and produces less hydrochloric acid. With people today taking antacids constantly because of improper eating, the risk of getting parasites keeps increasing. You can usually eliminate the use of antacids when you eat a proper balance of acid and alkaline foods. The practice of giving children antacids for the calcium content is just setting them up for parasite attack.

The incomplete digestion of proteins creates a number of problems for the body, including the development of allergies and the formation of toxic substances. Enzymes called proteases not only help to digest proteins, but serve other important functions such as keeping the small intestine free from parasites including yeast, protozoa, and intestinal worms. A lack of proteases or other digestive secretions greatly increases a person's risk of having intestinal infections.

Part of eating healthy is using good hygiene around the places you prepare and eat your food. The improper handling, preparation, and cooking of food is probably one of the main reasons people get parasites in the first place. Since foods can be the vehicle by which parasites enter our bodies, it is important to take the time and care to clean them of parasites along with chemicals, pesticides, fungi, bacteria, and other contaminants.

One of the most overlooked steps in food preparation is the proper washing of vegetables, fruits, eggs, legumes and grains. This also includes fish and meats. Removing as many toxins as possible may prevent adverse reactions and decrease the toxic load on the immune system and liver. Washing also helps to remove waxes, dirt, dust, and mold from the food's surface. Unless you use a good cleansing bath for all food, it is better to eliminate uncooked foods from the diet, and cook all animal flesh until well done.

When you arrive home after shopping at the grocery store, you can clean all your food at once. Fill the sink with about a gallon of pure filtered water. If you don't need a gallon of water to wash your foods, then reduce the amount of the water and the food wash accordingly. Use tap water if that is the only available water source. Add the food wash of your choice. Use a vegetable brush on the more sturdy vegetables and rub the other vegetables with your hands. When using a food spray instead of a bulk wash, you will need to spray your foods well, rub gently, and rinse well. The following are several methods for washing your food:

- Add 7 to 8 drops of liquid grapefruit seed extract to one gallon of water and use as your food wash. This excellent vegetable and fruit rinse can be bought at most health-food stores. Its potency as a bactericide and fungicide will help kill what is consuming, decaying, or contaminating your food. Various tests using grapefruit seed extract in low concentrations have extended the shelf or transport life of fruits and vegetables by as much as 400 percent. Buy the concentrated form.
- Dilute one tablespoon of 35 percent food-grade hydrogen peroxide in one gallon of water and wash all of your foods in this. Always use 35 percent food-grade hydrogen peroxide in a dilute solution. Never use it as a concentrate without diluting it first. To make a 3 percent solution, mix 1 ounce 35 percent food grade hydrogen peroxide with 11 ounces of distilled water. For pets (dogs and cats) use 1 ounce of 3 percent hydrogen peroxide to one quart of water.
- Dilute 2 ounces of freshly squeezed lemon juice, with rind included, in 1 gallon of pure filtered water and use this as your food wash.
- Buy a good food wash from your health-food store. There are several varieties available. See their instructions for use as a spray or as a bulk wash. Make sure this food wash will be adequate against parasites, as well as bacteria and viruses.
- Scrub all fruits and vegetables with a food-grade soap and water, then rinse well.

Into the food bath, place the fruits, vegetables, meat or fish to be treated. The thin-skinned fruits and leafy vegetables (berries, plums, lettuce) will require 15 minutes. The root vegetables and heavy-skinned fruits (apples and bananas) will require 30 minutes. Meats, foul, eggs, and fish need to soak for 20 minutes. Put each type of animal flesh in a different wash. Make a fresh wash for each group. Remove the food from the bath and place into a fresh water bath for another 10 to 15 minutes.

Regardless of what food wash you use, dry the food carefully, preferably with 100 percent cotton dish towels. Then wrap them in dry dish towels for storage to prevent moisture accumulation. Keeping foods in plastic or paper bags will shorten their shelf-life. Now, the food is ready to be put into storage.

There are several advantages to using this treatment. Fruits and vegetables will keep longer. The wilted ones will return to a fresh crispness. The faded color will vanish, and the jaded flavor will be gone. For your effort you will have fresh, crisp vegetables that will keep twice as long. The flavors will be greatly enhanced, tasting almost fresh picked from the garden.

Peeling root vegetables may remove some of the mold, but it also just spreads it around, so scrub before peeling. Clean melons before slicing them. When you cut into the melon the knife blade drags whatever is on the outside of the melon onto the flesh of the melon. The same applies to squash, pumpkin, avocado, oranges, etc.

Freeze beef and pork at minus 20° C for at least 24 hours. The minimum temperature that foods need to cooked to kill most parasites is 160° F. Use a meat thermometer to check the internal temperature of meats in several places. Eating any type of rare meat these days is not a good idea. You can cook beef at 160°, but pork, veal, and lamb need to have an internal temperature of 170° F. Be sure that the meat is well cooked in all parts. There are some cookwares that work to kill parasites at lower temperatures, but do not destroy the vitamins and minerals in the food. If you use a conventional oven, cook at a minimum of 325° F.

Freeze fish at a minus 18° C for at least 48 hours to kill larvae. Bake fish at 400° F for eight to ten minutes per inch of thickness, or until it is flaky and white. It is best to buy your seafood from established dealers rather than from roadside stands or trucks. When cooking fish or meat in a microwave oven it is important to note that a microwave oven tends to heat unevenly. Check the internal temperature of the meat in several different places. Heat fish to an internal temperature of 140° F for at least five minutes.

Clean and disinfect all cooking utensils, cutting boards, or surfaces that come in contact with uncooked foods. Do not sample unwashed foods before they are thoroughly cooked. Only eat raw fish that has been commercially blast-frozen. Ask if your fish market carries blast-frozen fish or try to find one that does.

CHAPTER 5

The Immune System's Role

A parasitic infection may be only one element in the much larger issue of a depressed immune system. In order to effectively defend ourselves against parasites, we also have to strengthen our immune system. The immune system is the first line of defense against infection. You invite opportunistic organisms into your body when your defense system is not strong and healthy. Despite the progress made in medicine, people are becoming more vulnerable to infection. Human bodies are getting weaker, while invading parasites, as well as bacteria, viruses, and fungi grow stronger.

Parasites are often difficult to diagnose and even more difficult to treat. The best solution is always prevention. Parasites are opportunistic. They live because our weakened immune defense system is taking a beating. The amount of chronic stressors makes us more susceptible. They include pollution, antibiotics and many other pharmaceutical drugs, pesticides and other chemical pollutants, alcohol, drug abuse, tobacco, emotional stress, fatigue, and poor diet.

Parasites, especially worms, activate the immune response. As the parasite continues to invade the body, it can damage areas including the gastrointestinal and nervous system. This creates further stress on an already weakened immune system. When there is continual assault and damage, it eventually leads to the exhaustion of the immune system. A weakened body cannot defend itself adequately. Each challenge to the immune system stimulates it into action until it is so exhausted that it fails to respond.

The same factors that increase our susceptibility to parasites also increases our susceptibility to cancer and other chronic illnesses. The increase of AIDS, chronic fatigue syndrome, lupus, and other immune related illnesses are a signal that our immune competence has become seriously impaired. A parasite infestation also gives off toxic byproducts that can trigger autoimmune reactions, or manifest as other diseases.

If you have ever had an acute parasitic infection you know how debilitating parasites' toxins can be. A chronic parasitic infection may produce few symptoms, but the low levels of toxins can create a constant burden on the immune system over a long period, making the body's ability to resist other organisms and infections less likely.

When you take an antibiotic that kills bacteria indiscriminately, both the good and the bad, it upsets the natural ecology of the body. This often leads to yeast overgrowth and the occurrence of *Trichomonas vaginalis,* a common parasite of the vaginal area. In some areas of the United States, this organism is one of the most commonly found. For those who are undergoing immune-suppressive drug therapies for cancer and organ transplants, the risk for a parasitic infestation is very high. The effects of parasites in healthy individuals may not produce any symptoms, while in immune-compromised patients it can be life-threatening.

Immune dysfunction can come from many different causes, yet the most perplexing is the involvement of the yeast, *Candida albicans.* This organism probably lives within most people and remains entirely compatible for an individual's lifetime. At any time it can establish itself in the tissues and release its byproducts into the bloodstream affecting the immune, endocrine, and nervous systems. It also appears to be a complicating factor in immune dysfunction, leaving the door open for parasites.

It should not be surprising that people who take good care of themselves have a stronger immune system than those who do not. To really help your immune system, you must change your eating habits and emphasize healthy, live foods. Undernourishment is generally regarded as the most frequent cause of a person's impaired immune system. Even marginal deficiencies of single or multiple nutrients can cause profound problems. Most of the people in this country fit this deficient nutritional picture. What you put into your body must be easily digested and assimilated, and not adding additional stress to the digestive system. Dealing with stress, whether it affects one's emotional, psychological, or biological processes, requires enzyme-rich balanced meals.

Immune system dysfunction often results from this combination of poor nutrition, chronic stress and various environmental pollutants. Of these three factors, poor nutrition is probably the most significant. Much of this country's susceptibility to disease, including parasites, is linked at least in part to dietary excesses and imbalances. The most harmful foods that you can eat are the wrong fats, dairy products, white flour, sugar and sugar substitutes, and meat injected with hormones, steroids, and antibiotics. Foods become even more dangerous when treated with pesticides. This all affects the immune system. Diet plays a vital role in regaining and maintaining health, and influences the immune system in many ways.

- Sugar and other refined and simple carbohydrates such as sucrose, fructose, honey, and concentrated fruit juice all reduce white blood cell production by 50 percent within 30 minutes of ingestion. This impaired immunity can last for over five hours. Most Americans consume 150 grams of sucrose, including other refined simple sugars daily, and may be suffering from a chronic weakened immune system as a result.
- The consistent eating of allergy-causing foods impairs the immune system. Test for food allergies and other sensitivities.
- The over-consumption of caffeine reduces levels of immunoglobulins in the serum. These globulins are a necessary part of the immune response.
- The development of intestinal toxins weakens the immune response and impairs digestion.
- Malabsorption, as a result of diarrhea, irritable bowel syndrome, intestinal food allergies, intestinal infection, or bacterial flora imbalances, impairs the immune system and increase stress.
- A lack of adequate calories, especially protein intake, will dramatically decrease the body's ability to cope with stress. This type of malnutrition impairs immunity in general.
- Obesity is associated with decreased immune status. Cholesterol and triglycerides levels are usually elevated in obese people. When these levels are too high, it impairs their immune system.

Sleeping eight hours daily is essential for most working adults. Daily therapeutic relaxation is also an essential component. Allow yourself to re-experience inner peace and poise daily with meditation, prayer, chanting, listening to peaceful music without distraction or interruptions, or having a quiet bath to candlelight.

The ability to manage stress is profoundly affected and controlled by a person's mental attitude. Negative and pessimistic thinking creates stress while a positive change in attitude reduces stress. When a person is stressed, especially if it is chronic, the digestive system begins to get less blood, oxygen, and nutrition, as does the immune system. It results in impaired nutrition and leads to an increased risk of infection and illness.

What about the connection between allergies and parasites? When a change in a person's lifestyle causes them to be less exposed to parasites, the immune system starts to respond to other substances that can be nontoxic. Eric Ottensen, head of the Clinical Parasitology Section at the National Institute of Allergy and Infectious Disease in Bethesda, Maryland, says this is because the specific immune response to parasites is affected by immunoglobulins E (IgE), which are usually involved in allergic responses to inhalants such as pollens and dust. When people reduce their contact with parasites through properly prepared and cooked foods and other measures, the IgE immune reaction remains activated. It then directs its attention to otherwise harmless factors. Then, suddenly, there is an allergy.

In one study, the antibody IgE was detected in 16 out of 27 carriers of intestinal parasites. IgEs were also detected in 236 out of 312 food-sensitive people. Although IgE plays a role in the expulsion of intestinal parasites in experimental animals, its overall contribution to our defense remains a subject of controversy. So if you test positive for IgEs in your blood, do you have a food allergy, a parasite, or both?

Recently developed is a natural boost to the immune system called "transfer factors." Transfer factors are small immune messenger molecules that transfer immune recognition signals between immune cells and assist in educating naive immune cells to the presence of danger. This communication occurs within the immune system.

Transfer factors has the unique ability to trigger our most sophisticated immune system mechanism while also having antiparasitic properties. It is the main immune system chemical in a mother's first milk (colostrum), and is the first shield against infection and disease. Only recently was it discovered that colostrum contains other immune system messengers with the most important being transfer factors. Your immune system provides constant surveillance of the entire body to make sure that only the cells that are supposed to be there are there. It is the first to recognize alien substances such as bacteria, viruses, parasites, or other foreign substances and immediately plans an attack.

It not only reacts to each invading pathogen, but remembers the invader and quickly acts upon future invasions with an overwhelming response. The immune system uses hormone-like signal substances to communicate between cells. This is where the substance called transfer factors becomes so valuable. For people whose immunity is not up to par, it can transfer an apparently mature immune response within 24 hours. It is equally effective whether given by injection or taken orally. It has been shown that long-term oral ingestion of transfer factor preparations is safe. The elderly and children are especially at risk for infections, including parasites.

Fortunately the diligence of persistent researchers, Dr. Gary Wilson and Dr. Greg Paddock, has won USDA approval of their patented transfer factor technology. This technology has the potential to help us in the fight against many conditions that threaten our health and weaken our immune system. Transfer factor could have the potential of managing or eliminating the illness caused by many parasites. As you have heard or read in the news lately, many bacteria, viruses, and even parasites have become resistant to the latest drugs. The scope of the situation may become enormous. The medicines that have helped us in the past may be of no value in the future. Meanwhile, the "super bugs" are getting stronger.

Trichomonas vaginalis is just one of the pathogens that have become resistant to antibiotics. So have many of the organisms that cause malaria. Some protozoa, such as cryptosporidium, are not affected by antibiotics either. The difference between people getting over infections from these organisms, or not, is the strength of their immune system. There is a good chance that you have been exposed to parasites such as crytosporidium, since it is in many of the drinking water systems in this country. Studies published in *Infection and Immunity*, 1993, have shown that the immune factors in colostrum are able to ameliorate or eliminate the clinical symptoms of those suffering from this protozoa. Other parasites affected by transfer factors are the blood flukes and the parasite that causes cutaneous leishmaniasis.

As long as your immune system is strong and protects you, there is little concern about severe illness from cryptosporidium. But considering that most Americans eat a junk-food diet and suffer from various chronic stressors, they don't have adequate immune function to protect them against these invaders. As we get older our immune system gradually weakens, unless special effort is made to strengthen it. The conditions of close contact with others and diminished personal hygiene have led to more cases of confirmed infections.

The emerging food and water-borne diseases are increasing at a staggering rate. In any type of disease, it would be helpful to have a rapid onset remedy to help people from either getting sick or lessen the effects if they have already contracted an infection. Since transfer factor has a quick onset, it may be the most effective way of dealing with pathogens. Since it is also nontoxic, there would not be the side effects experienced from taking drugs or even some of the herbs available to fight parasites. This substance may have the ability to arm the immune system and keep it more vigilant.

Recent research confirms that improved nutrition can have a profound effect on the immune system. Various vitamins, minerals and nutritional factors improve the performance of the immune system. Many of the water soluble vitamins including vitamin C, bioflavonoids, and the B vitamins. In addition, the adrenal glands need to be supported during stressful situations when the body is more susceptible to disease conditions.

The fat-soluble vitamins, such as vitamin A (or beta carotene) and vitamin E, are antioxidant nutrients that protect cellular constituents from damaging effects often caused by pollutants. They also stimulate the immune system by causing an increase in the performance of the immune response against parasites.

Selenium and zinc are important trace minerals to the function of the immune system. They help to improve the function of the thymus gland and produce enzymes that prevent oxidation. Many people do not get enough of these minerals in their diet. The thymus is the major gland of our immune system. It is responsible for the production of T lymphocytes, a type of white blood cell responsible for resistance to infections such as parasites. Perhaps the most widely used herb for enhancing our immune system is *Echinacea angustifolia*. This herb has a profound immune enhancing effect especially for the thymus gland. Other helpful herbs include *Glycyrrhiza glabra* (licorice) and *Viscum album* (European mistletoe).

Arginine is a nonessential amino acid produced in the body that enhances immune function. It also increases the size and activity of the thymus gland and aids in liver detoxification by neutralizing ammonia, a waste product of parasites. Taking 500 mg of arginine each morning reduces the parasite's toxic effects.

Ornithine is another nonessential amino acid that is manufactured in the body from arginine. It also improves the function of the immune system and liver. It detoxifies any ammonia produced by parasites. Take two 500 mg tablets of ornithine at bedtime on the first night of treatment (according to Dr. Hulda Clark), increase the ornithine dosage to four tablets the second night, six tablets the third night, and reduce the dosage to four tablets the fourth night.

The lymphatic system plays a large part in draining waste products from tissues and filtering this waste from the body. It can be improved by increasing the circulation through regular exercise and proper breathing. The herbs that improve lymph function are *Hydrastis canadensis* (goldenseal), *Echinacea angustifolia* (echinacea), and *Panax ginseng* (Korean ginseng).

The spleen is the largest mass of lymphatic tissue in the body. It enhances the immune function by secreting compounds that may benefit people with parasites such as the ones that causes malaria. Goldenseal may improve spleen function through its ability to increase blood flow as well as increase the activity of the white blood cells called macrophages. These are the cells that attack and kill many types of parasites.

The liver produces the majority of lymph in the body even though it is not considered a lymphatic organ. Some of the cells present in the liver are responsible for filtering toxic foreign compounds absorbed from the gastrointestinal tract. Periodically, cleanse the liver by drinking the juice of a fresh lemon in a cup of very warm water. This should be done first thing in the morning. It is important to give your liver support especially during detoxification programs. Daily use of milk thistle extract during these programs insures normal liver clearance of toxins as well as protection of the liver cells. The recommended dosage of milk thistle extract standardized to 70 percent silymarin content is 200 mg. three times daily. With improvement, the dosage may be reduced to 200 mg. twice daily. This lower dosage may also be used for preventive purposes or as part of a cleansing and detoxification program. Milk thistle extract is virtually without any side effects and may be used by a wide range of people including pregnant and lactating women. It can cause a mild, transient laxative effect in some people.

CHAPTER 6

What Parasites Are Feeding On You?

There are two major categories of parasites. One category consists of microscopic parasites that consist mainly of protozoa. Protozoa function similarly to bacteria by traveling through the bloodstream to most parts of the human body. Microscopic parasites do not live off their host as such, but can thrive on processed foods. Their excretion can cause serious problems within the human body. They reproduce without laying eggs, but by duplicating themselves. Most protozoan infections run their course without too many complications in a person with a healthy immune system.

The other category consists of large parasites, primarily worms. These worm types are often large enough to be seen without the aid of a microscope. They can grow from several inches long up to several feet. Eggs are deposited in the intestinal tract where they stick to the walls of the intestines and hatch, allowing the young worms to feed on the food that the host eats. In some species of worms, the eggs pass out of the body before they hatch. It is outside they eventually grow into adults and the process is repeated.

Usually, worms do not travel to other parts of the body other than the digestive tract. There are worms that exist in other countries that have the ability to burrow out of the digestive tract into other organs. This is usually not the case in the United States, but we are seeing other types of worms being brought into this country more and more. When a worm infestation is present, intervention is almost always required.

The parasites referred to in this book are specifically protozoa (single-celled organisms) and worms (multi-celled organisms) that invade and feed off their host. Parasites have been coevolving with humans for a long time and their presence in the body does not serve any known good purpose for the host. Illness often results when these disease-promoting organisms are ingested from contaminated food and water supplies. There are parasites that can also infect the skin or enter the bloodstream through insect bites. They can deplete the body of essential nutrients and overwhelm the immune system leading to serious illness and even death. There are four different groups of parasitic invaders being discussed at length in this book: they are the single-cell protozoa, tapeworms, roundworms, and flukes.

I. PROTOZOA

A. Amebas
Blastocystis hominis
Endolimax nana
Entamoeba histolytica

B. Ciliates
Balantidium coli

C. Flagellates
Dientamoeba fragilis
Giardia lamblia
Leishmania tropica
Trichomonas vaginalis

D. Microspordia (Blood Parasites)
Plasmodium falciparum
Trypanosoma cruzi

E. Coccidia (Tissue Parasites)
Cryptosporidium parvum
Toxoplasma gondii

Cyclospora cayetanensis (unknown classification)

II. WORMS OR HELMINTHS

A. Cestodes or Tapeworms

Dipylidium caninum (dog tapeworm)
Diphyllobothrium latum (fish tapeworm)
Hymenolepsis nana (dwarf tapeworm)
Taenia saginata (beef tapeworm)
Taenia solium (pork tapeworm)

B. Nematodes or Roundworms

Ancylostoma caninum (hookworm)
Anisakis simplex (fish roundworm)
Ascaris lumbricoides (giant intestinal roundworm)
Dirofilaria immitis (dog heartworm)
Enterobium vernicularis (pinworm or seatworm)
Eustrongylides spp. (fish roundworm)
Necator americanus/Ancylostoma duodenale (hookworm)
Strongyloides stercoralis (threadworm)
Toxocara canis/cati (dog and cat roundworms)
Trichinella spiralis (pork roundworm)
Trichostrongylus (herbivore roundworm)
Trichuris trichiura (whipworm)

C. Trematodes or Flukes

Clonorchis sinensis (liver flukes)
Fasciolopsis buski (intestinal fluke)
Nanophyetus spp. (fish flu flukes)
Paragonimus westermani (lung flukes)
Schistosoma spp. (blood flukes)

Protozoans

Protozoans are a group of single-celled, usually microscopic organisms, that have the ability to reproduce rapidly in the intestinal tract of their host, and migrate to other organs and tissues, or to red blood cells. They are capable of infecting every tissue in the body. When protozoans infect the intestines of humans, they may be the unsuspected cause of chronic illness and fatigue. Most of them are transmitted through fecal contaminated food and impure water. Protozoans are also carried by insects such as the mosquitoes that harbor the malaria organism. These parasites may remain active in the body for a person's entire lifetime, causing multiple complications and revisitations, such as with malarial fever.

Contaminated water is a significant problem because when protozoans are in their cyst phase, they are not necessarily killed by the use of chlorine in the drinking water. This is because some protozoans produce a closed sac called a cyst that allows them safe passage through water or food. This cyst phase also allows them to move through the digestive enzymes and through the digestive tract of their host to the small intestine. This would normally kill the adult protozoan. Parasitic protozoans, such as *Giardia lamblia*, then travel into the large intestine where they feed, grow, and begin to reproduce. The spread of protozoans in our bodies can cause abscesses in the liver, lungs, heart, and brain. Virulent strains can even be dangerous to our health and result in fatal dysentery.

Usually non-virulent strains predominate in the United States, but even these can cause severe diarrhea in those with a weakened immune system. Lately, the frequency of intestinal infections caused by the ameba, *Entamoeba histolytica,* or by the flagellated *Giardia lamblia,* is alarming many public health officials. It has become prevalent throughout the United States with at least 7 million people infected. It seems that protozoan infections are alive and well, and not just in under-developed countries where sanitary conditions are poor.

Being infected with some type of protozoan is an accepted way of life in many parts of the world. It is estimated that one fifth of the world's population is infected by protozoans. One of the ways that these organisms move around the world is by troops during wars entering areas where protozoans are commonly found, making it difficult to avoid contamination. The soldiers then carry the parasite back to their homeland, often showing no symptoms unless they have a compromised immune system. It usually takes several months longer to treat protozoan infection, such as giardia and cryptosporidium, than it does to treat an infestation of worms.

Worldwide, *Giardia lamblia* is probably the fourth most prevalent human intestinal parasite following *Blastocystis hominis, Entamoeba histolytica,* and *Cryptosporidium parvum.* A recent study at John Hopkins Hospital found that 18 percent of a randomly selected group of blood samples showed a past or present infection of the parasite *Giardia lamblia.*

Some of the better labs request several different ways to collect specimens for the best recovery of organisms. The lab will find larvae, cysts, or eggs in the stools, but it may require up to six different stool specimens to make a positive diagnosis. Collection of the stool specimens may need to be done over the course of several days or weeks. Blood (serologic) tests are also done by some labs. A biopsy is definitive with intestinal lesions. If there is a liver abscess, it can possibly be seen on x-ray, radioisotopic liver scan, or an ultrasound scan. Other tests may be necessary.

Parasitic protozoans belong to five groups: ameba, flagellates, ciliates, coccidia (tissue parasites), and microspordia (blood parasites). They are called amebas because of their ability to change forms, flagellates because they have a whip-like appendage for movement, ciliates because of their rhythmic sweeping movements, coccidia because they are inside tissues and cells.

BALANTIDIUM COLI

Balantidium coli is the largest intestinal protozoan found in humans and the only pathogen that has cilia, causing it to have rhythmic sweeping movements. It is found worldwide and causes the disease "balantidiasis." The life cycle is similar to the ameba *Entamoeba histolytica*. The cysts of this parasite are transmitted by food and water contaminated with pig and occasionally monkey feces. Person to person transmission usually involves food handlers. Infection is rare in humans but may reach 100 percent in pigs where it is nonpathogenic.

Infections in humans are usually without symptoms. When symptoms do occur they are usually self-limiting and include diarrhea, abdominal pain, and inflammation of the colon. Occasional there is constipation, anorexia, weakness, insomnia, and weight loss. If there is any ulceration of the intestinal wall of the colon, it can extend to the liver and occasionally it is transported by the blood into the spinal fluid. Opportunistic bacteria could grow where the intestinal wall is ulcerated. This protozoan has been associated with chronic fatigue syndrome. This organism usually lives in the large intestine where it can invade and destroy the wall lining. In severe infections, it is possible to have such a bad case of dysentery that it will cause death.

A stool or tissue sample can be examined microscopically for cysts or larvae. It is more likely to find the cysts in normal stool and the larvae in diarrhea. The oral administration of the drugs oxytetracycline, iodoquinol, diidohydroxyquin, metronidazole is commonly used to treat this organism. Sometimes the antibiotic, tetracycline, is included. Prevention and control are generally similar to those used for any amebic infection. Good sanitation and personal hygiene are the best ways to reduce this parasite.

BLASTOCYSTIS HOMINIS

The Institute of Parasitic Diseases (IPD) did a study and found that half of the people tested had *Blastocystis hominis*. It was found in more stool specimens than any other parasite. Infections are more frequent in adult males and in immune compromised people with chronic fatigue syndrome. It may take repeated or long term exposure in order to establish an infection. There is not a cyst or larvae stage as usually found in the typical protozoan. This organism infects the intestines where the small intestine meets the colon. It is hard to eradicate because of its ability to lodge itself in the wall of the intestine.

In some healthy individuals this parasite does not cause any symptoms. Other people suffer from gastrointestinal illness when it is present. It seems that *Blastocystis hominis* is probably a weak pathogen in those people whose overall health is compromised. Also, different strains of this organism are more pathogenic than others. Canadian strains are usually nonpathogenic while those of some Middle Eastern countries appear to cause illness. *Blastocystis hominis* was just as often found in people with symptoms as those without symptoms. Studies have compared *Blastocystis hominis* to pathogens such as *Entamoeba histolytica* and *Giardia lamblia,* which are frequently shed in low numbers and found in a considerable number of individuals who do not show any symptoms.

This organism can suppress the immune system and cause acute gastrointestinal symptoms when present in large numbers or in weakened individuals. The symptoms could include abdominal pain or cramps, nausea, vomiting, gas, diarrhea, fever, sleeplessness, dizziness, and fatigue. It is also associated with more chronic conditions such as inflammatory bowel disease. It is rare to have a report of symptoms associated outside the intestinal tract, but it has been found in the fluid of an inflamed knee joint. Other symptoms include weight loss, headaches, allergies, nervous disorders, itchiness, and muscle problems. The toxic byproducts from this parasite can lead to autoimmune reactions.

When *Blastocystis hominis* exists with other weak pathogens it has been implicated in several chronic conditions including irritable bowel disease, chronic fatigue syndrome, and different forms of arthritis. People who are infected only with *Blastocystis hominis*, as well as those infected at the same time with *Entamoeba* species often experience a number of symptoms. The most frequent ones are bloating, diarrhea, flatulence, constipation, cramps, and malabsorption.

This parasite may be even more common, but due to poor laboratory techniques it is often not detected. When using more sophisticated laboratory techniques, then *Blastocystis hominis* is found in more of the specimens examined and is one of the most commonly detected parasites in stool samples at the Great Smokies Diagnostic Laboratory. On a blood test there may be an increase in a particular white blood cell call eosinophils due to being infected with this parasite. The drugs of choice are metronidazole or iodoquinol.

CRYPTOSPORIDIUM PARVUM

Cryptosporidium parvum was not considered to be a health risk for humans as recently as 1993, when people in Milwaukee, Wisconsin, became ill with diarrhea after drinking contaminated drinking water. This tiny parasite is a single cell, microscopic animal that can infect a human's digestive tract and cause severe gastrointestinal disease. The infective stage of this organism, the oocyst, is about half the size of a red blood cell. Less than 10 organisms can cause an infection. Humans can be infected at any time in their lives, but only previous exposure to the parasite results in either full or partial immunity.

The life cycle begins in humans with the ingestion of the oocyst. This is the resistant stage found in the environment. The preferred site of infection is the last part of the small intestine, where it can penetrate individual skin cells. Multiple divisions occur until the parasite reaches a phase where it can reproduce itself indefinitely. A resistant wall (cyst phase) is formed around some of them in one part of its life cycle and passed out with the stool into the environment.

Each generation can develop and mature in as little as 12-14 hours. Because of its rapid life cycle, plus its ability to reinfect its host, huge numbers of organisms can colonize the intestinal tract in several days. When the lower part of the small intestine becomes too crowded, the parasite often moves to other locations, such as higher up in the small intestines or further down to the large intestine. In people with a suppressed immune system, cryptosporidium can sometimes be found in the stomach, the ducts of the liver and pancreas, and the respiratory tract.

The disease caused by cryptosporidium is spread by putting something in the mouth that has been contaminated with the feces of an infected person or animal. You can also be infected by drinking contaminated water or eating raw or undercooked food contaminated with the cysts (an egg-like form of the parasite that is the infectious stage) or hand-to-mouth transfer of cysts from surfaces that may have become contaminated with microscopic amounts of feces. It is possible to acquire cryptosporidium from any food touched by a contaminated food handler. Fertilizing salad vegetables with manure is another possible source of human infection.

Outbreaks since 1984 in the United States and Canada have been associated with day care centers and directly related to the changing of diapers. Childcare workers and the diaper-aged children who attend these centers are at an increased risk of infection. Larger outbreaks are usually due to a contaminated water supply. One parasite specialty laboratory looked at 66 different filtered water treatment plants in 14 states. What they found was that 27 percent of the collected samples contained cryptosporidium cysts.

Other ways to acquire this parasite is exposure to human feces by sexual contact, and caregivers who might come in direct contact with feces while caring for an infected person at home or in a medical facility. Once infected, anyone with a suppressed immune system, such as chemotherapy patients, is at a very high risk for severe illness.

Cryptosporidium is widespread in the environment and can be found in lakes and streams. In North America, March through June is the time of year when cryptosporidium becomes a problem in surface waters in most areas when spring rains increase run-off. This is also a time when many young animals are present in the environment to pass numbers of oocysts. Cows, pigs, cats, dogs, and other mammals may contribute to the increased numbers of this parasite in rural and urban areas. It is nearly impossible to determine all origins of cryptosporidium infection. This is a parasite that can be acquired from public water supplies or transmitted to humans by companion animals, such as kittens and puppies, or by contact with other humans.

Cryptosporidium may be one of those underreported causes of illness because most people don't think they are infected with a parasite when they get sick. They assume it is some type of influenza with diarrhea and abdominal cramps. Symptoms can appear from two to ten days after being infected. In otherwise healthy people, the symptoms usually last one to two weeks before the immune system is able to stop the infection. In some outbreaks at day care centers, diarrhea can last 1–4 weeks. The symptoms produced could include headaches, nausea, vomiting, and a low-grade fever.

Even though cryptosporidium may cause a self-limited diarrhea in adults, it can be the cause of major diarrhea in children. The elderly and very young are especially at risk and can become critical much faster than the rest of the population. The nature of an acute intestinal disease is characterized by severe watery diarrhea, but may also be without symptoms. If a person has a suppressed immune system as usually seen with AIDS, or a recent organ or bone marrow transplant, then a cryptosporidium infection may become chronic and life-threatening. Gastrointestinal symptoms may become severe with overwhelming watery diarrhea and marked intestinal injury. AIDS patients may have the disease for life with the severe watery diarrhea contributing to death.

Lung and trachea infections in humans that are caused by cryptosporidium are associated with coughing and frequently a low-grade fever. These symptoms are often accompanied by severe intestinal distress. For the most part, lung infections are confined to those who are immune deficient. However, an infant can have a perfectly normal immune system, but get sicker if there is also a virus present at the same time. The virus lowered the child's resistance. Invasion of the lung area may also be fatal.

This is a parasite that makes little effort to evade the immune system of its host. Its success appears to be because of its ability to develop rapidly and flood the environment with its oocysts. If this parasite was not so effectively eliminated from the body, it would quickly kill its host through dehydration and electrolyte imbalance.

No one really knows how many oocysts it takes to establish an infection in humans. One study suggested that the infectious dose in humans could be anywhere from 30 to 132. Another study, using more aggressive organisms, suggests that even lower numbers of oocysts can sometimes cause disease. Individuals certainly seem to have various degrees of susceptibility to this parasite.

In some places such as Brazil, this parasite was present in 25 percent of the people with AIDS. Other surveys indicate that about 2 percent of the population in North America have this parasite. Blood test surveys indicate that 80 percent of the population has been infected at one time or another with this parasite.

In January of 1997, an outbreak of cryptosporidium occurred after drinking apple cider. In September of 1996, there was an outbreak associated with eating home-made chicken salad. In May of 1995, a non-food outbreak of cryptosporidium occurred in a day-camp. In September of 1995, the Minnesota Department of Health received reports of acute abdominal problems among an estimated 50 attendees at a social event.

As mentioned earlier, one of the largest outbreaks of cryptosporidium, in 1993, infected half of the population of Milwaukee, Wisconsin. This tiny parasite became immune to the chlorine, and infested the drinking water. Dozens died after drinking the contaminated water. It is not generally fatal unless you have a compromised immune system. It caused chronic diarrhea that lingered for weeks. The eggs were so small that many of them slipped through the water filtering system. Since that event, other large cities have found cryptosporidium in their water system, such as San Francisco and New York City. During 1987, a waterborne outbreak in Georgia produced illness in approximately 13,000 individuals. Cryptosporidium infection should be considered whenever there is a suspected food-borne illness.

In third-world countries, the prevalence is even higher. It is thought that up to 70 percent of the people may have been exposed to this pathogen. In AIDS patients, the numbers of individuals suffering from chronic illness from this parasite are thought to be about 10 percent in industrialized nations and up to 40 percent in some third world countries.

The various laboratories performing diagnostic testing on cryptosporidium cysts in the water have varying degrees of accuracy. Since the routine stool examination used for most parasites usually fails to detect cryptosporidium, a stool specimen should be examined using tests available especially for this parasite. A commercial kit is available that uses fluorescent antibody. Diagnosis has also been made by biopsy and staining the organism.

You can prevent this parasite by avoiding water or food that may be contaminated. Wash your hands after using the toilet and before handling food. If you work in a childcare facility be sure to wash your hands thoroughly with plenty of warm, soapy water after every diaper change, even if you wear gloves. As a caregiver, you should wash your hands after bathing patients, emptying bedpans, changing soiled linen, or otherwise coming in contact with the stools of patients. If you have been infected with this organism, wash your hands often to prevent spreading the disease to other people around you.

During community-wide outbreaks caused by contaminated drinking water, boil the drinking water for one minute to kill the cryptosporidium parasite. The cysts are resistant to most chemical disinfectants, but are susceptible to drying and the ultraviolet portion of sunlight. Ultraviolet radiation is being used in some water purifiers to kill this organism. An effective therapy appears to be in maintaining a healthy, intact immune system. The drug, spiramycin, has had some success and paromomycin sulfate (humatin) appears to have promise. This organism may be affected by metronidazole followed by iodoquinol. Other drugs used include octreotide or aflornithine.

HIV-infected people should avoid drinking potentially contaminated water such as water from lakes or rivers, and exposure unpasteurized milk or milk products, and avoid exposure to farm animals and places where these animals are raised. Wash hands after contact with pets, and wash hands after gardening or other contact with soil. Avoid any sexual activity that brings you in contact with the feces of an infected partner. It is very important to follow safe sex guidelines.

If you suspect that you have been infected, see your physician. It is important for persons with a poorly functioning immune system to seek medical attention early in the course of their disease. People who have normal immune systems improve without taking antibiotic or antiparasitic medications. Drink plenty of fluids and get extra rest. Physicians may prescribe medication to slow the diarrhea during recovery. Supportive therapy is a basic and necessary part of treatment. Discontinuing immune suppressive chemotherapy will help to restore proper immune function and help to resolve the intestinal infection in some people.

CYCLOSPORA CAYETANENSIS

Cyclospora is a parasite found primarily in human feces. It was found in Guatemalan raspberries that spread illness to over 1000 people. Prior to this outbreak, the three minor outbreaks reported in the United States had all been traced to using water contaminated by human fecal waste. The carrier has not yet been discovered for cyclospora.

Usually, when we think of food poisoning, we think of eating undercooked meat, not wholesome fruits and vegetables. Finding contaminated produce is far from new. Lettuce, cantaloupe, and fresh apple cider have been blamed for illnesses caused by bacteria. With the contaminated raspberry scare, the public has started to question the quality of produce sold in the United States. The Center for Disease Control says that all past outbreaks of cyclospora are linked to tainted water and they don't believe that the raspberries were the original source of contamination.

Cyclospora can cause diarrhea, cramps, headaches, weight loss, decreased appetite, vomiting, fatigue, flatulence, bloating, itching skin, fever, and muscle aches. This parasite can also cause the chronic symptoms of malabsorption, anorexia, depression, and fibromyalgia. Some people with cyclospora do not have any symptoms and are unaware that they are harboring this parasite. Most protozoa are affected by metronidazole followed by iodoquinol; other drugs used are paromomylin or diloxanide furoate.

DIENTAMOEBA FRAGILIS

Dientamoeba fragilis is a parasite of the large intestine in humans. This pathogenic flagellate is considered one of the most frequent parasitic infections, especially in day care centers and other urban areas. It does not have a cyst stage in its life cycle so it lives in the intestinal tract, the cecum, and colon as a larva (trophozoite). This makes laboratory detection difficult. Unfortunately, many infected people go undetected.

Dientamoeba fragilis is transmitted by direct ingestion of the larvae (trophozoite). It can also be found within the eggs of some worms, especially pinworms. Infection with this parasite can cause diarrhea and abdominal discomfort. Their presence can lead to the development of chronic symptoms and lead to autoimmune reactions. Since it lives without a cyst stage, laboratory detection is difficult with stool samples. In the larva stage it is similar to an ameba. The drugs of choice are iodoquinol and paromomycin.

ENDOLIMAX NANA

The smallest of the intestinal amebas has recently become a pathogen. The larvae of *Endolimax nana* are small and move sluggishly in contrast to the rapid movements of *Entamoeba histolytica*. This ameba lives in the lower bowel, but has the ability to travel to other parts of the body. There are several references that say that rheumatoid arthritis is caused by *Endolimax nana,* as well as causing other collagen-related diseases. It has been associated with hives and reactive arthritis. The drug of choice is metronidazole with diiodohydroxyquine.

ENTAMOEBA HISTOLYTICA

Amoebiasis was defined in 1969 by the World Health Organization (WHO) as a condition in which a person is harboring the organism, *Entamoeba histolytica,* in the bowel. Theoretically, the ingestion of one viable cyst can cause an infection even if the person shows no clinical symptoms of the disease. It is estimated that this organism infects 400 million people in the world. The precise factors that make it a pathogen are not completely understood. *Entamoeba histolytica* can cause a life-threatening parasitic disease, with mortality world-wide second only to malaria.

This is a single celled parasitic ameba that infects predominantly humans and other primates. First there is the infective cyst phase that develops into the next stage in the small intestine. Once it reaches the small intestine, this parasite is satisfied to grow and multiply in the open spaces of the bowel, where it feeds on bacteria, tissue, or blood cells. It can penetrate the wall of the intestine where stool is stagnant. With diarrhea, the fragile larva passes unchanged in the liquid stool and rapidly dies upon exposure to room temperatures. If diarrhea is not present, the organisms usually develop into a cyst before leaving the bowels. The cysts survive outside the host in water and soil and on foods, especially under moist conditions.

They can spread from person to person through food or water or they can spread indirectly through fecal-oral contact, and by direct contact with dirty hands or objects, and by sexual contact. Dogs and cats can become infected, but usually do not shed cysts in their feces that would survive in the environment. So they are not the ones that contribute significantly to the transmission of this parasite.

It is found in poor countries where proper hygiene might be expected to be lax. But it is also found in this country's day care centers where post-potty hand washing isn't monitored, or in suburbs where wells are drilled too close to septic tanks. The infection spreads with the practice of anal-oral sex or indirectly from contaminated food eaten by travelers. In the United States the spread is usually person-to-person and the infection rate has been reported to be as much as 5 percent of the population. Most people that tested positive recently traveled to areas such as Mexico, or were exposed to unsanitary food handling.

People with chronic symptoms and people who carry the parasite, but without symptoms, are the most common sources of transmitting this parasite. Acutely ill people infested with invasive amebas are not significant transmitters since they usually pass the non-infective phase in their diarrhea. Flies and roaches are vectors that aid the spread of *Entamoeba histolytica*. Other factors associated with increased incidence of infection include being institutionalized or having had colonic irrigation using improperly sterilized equipment. All people are believed to be susceptible to infection, but anyone with a damaged or undeveloped immunity may suffer more severe forms of the disease. AIDS/ARC patients are very vulnerable. In recent times, food handlers are suspected of causing many scattered infections, but there has been no single large outbreak.

The onset of symptoms is highly variable. It is thought that the absence of symptoms or their intensity varies with such factors as the ameba strain, the immune health of the host, and associated bacteria or viruses. The ameba's enzymes help it to penetrate and digest human tissues. It also secretes toxic substances that probably contribute to the host's symptoms. You can be considered healthy and still harbor this parasite. In most cases, particularly in the temperate zones, the organism is not a pathogen and can live in the bowels as part of the normal bowel flora.

If there are any symptoms, diarrhea, flatulence, and abdominal pain with cramps, are the most frequent complaints. The diarrhea can come and go, alternating with episodes of normal stool or constipation over a period of months to years. Usually, the stools consist of one to four loose to watery, foul-smelling passages that contain mucus and blood. There may be tenderness in the abdominal area, liver, and colon. There can also be vague digestive distress, and include distention and bloating, weight loss, and fatigue. Most infections occur in the digestive tract, but other tissues may be invaded such as the liver by the spread of *Entamoeba histolytica* through the blood system. Complications of this disease include ulceration and abscesses, but intestinal blockage is rarely seen. Disease from this ameba can last for years.

A more severe form of infection, usually only seen in the tropics, is amebic dysentery. This disease has frequent fluid or semifluid stools often containing blood, mucus flecks, occasionally with a slight fever. There may be emaciation and anemia that can worsen between attacks. Severe ulceration of the gastrointestinal wall occurs in less than 16 percent of cases. In fewer cases, the parasite invades the soft tissues, most commonly the liver. Only rarely are masses formed that lead to intestinal obstruction. Bacterial infections may complicate the disease if the immune system is depressed in the host. Fatalities are infrequent. The symptoms can present with symptoms that make it difficult to differentiate from inflammatory bowel disease such as Crohn's disease and ulcerative colitis.

Entamoeba hartmanni is usually an organism that lives within us without causing many problems. Infected people usually only have one of the following symptoms: bloating, cramps, diarrhea, flatulence, or irritable bowel. Other symptoms could include allergies, nausea, nerve system and skin disorders, pain, and respiratory difficulties. *Entamoeba hartmanni* and *Entamoeba histolytica* may be interchangeable forms associated with various illnesses and stresses. It has been observed that people treated for *Entamoeba histolytica* retest positive with *Entamoeba hartmanni* a few weeks later.

Another common species of ameba is found in the mouth area, *Entamoeba gingivalis*. It is found in the area between the teeth and gums and around the jaw bones, eating away at these areas causing a variety of mouth disorders.

In heavy infections, the motile form (the trophozoite) can be seen in fresh feces. They are usually found in liquid or very soft stools while the cysts usually occur more frequently in formed stools. Even though human cases of infection are diagnosed by finding cysts shed with the stool, not every sample of stool has detectable cyst. So it is important to get multiple stool specimens—at least three—but it may take seven to confirm a positive diagnosis. Sometimes it takes intervals of several days between samples to get a positive parasite sample. Blood tests exist for chronic infections. If this protozoa is living in the liver, it may not be found in stool specimens.

Filtration is probably the most practical method for recovery from drinking water and liquid foods. There are many falsely negative results in some lab tests.

There is some evidence that a curative treatment for this ameba may make the host resistant to subsequent invasive amebas possibly by the production of antibodies. There is a high rate of infection with *Entamoeba histolytica* in immune compromised people compared to others who have adequate immune system function. Since the 1960s, antibiotic-resistant strains have been emerging. The cysts are very resistant to certain chemicals and can survive up to 72 hours in a chlorine solution routinely used in public water supplies. They can also survive in water for up to one month and temperatures up to 122° F.

The drug of choice is metronidazole (flagyl) followed by iodoquinol. Asymptomatic carriers are treated with iodoquinol or paromomycin. Emetine hydrochloride, dehydroemetine, chloroquine, diidohydroxyquin (diodoquin), diloxanide furoate (furamide), or tetracyclines are also used depending on the severity of the illness, location and dissemination of the infection.

GIARDIA LAMBLIA

This is a parasite that is seen worldwide It is found throughout this country infecting an estimated 18 million people and is increasing so rapidly that it may now be the most frequently found parasite. Some tested day-care centers found out that 99 percent of the children attending had a positive stool for *Giardia lamblia*. Susceptibility to infection depends on several factors: the virulence of the organism, and whether the immune system is functioning adequately. Giardia cysts are resistant to destruction by stomach acid in the host, especially if the amount is already inadequate. A healthy adult can acquire some protective immunity.

This is a single-celled protozoan, sometimes referred to as *Lamblia intestinalis* in Europe. Infection with giardia, called "giardiasis," is the most frequent cause of nonbacterial water-borne diarrhea in North America. Cool moist conditions favor the survival of this organism. The cyst is the survival form in the environment and infective stage of the organism. Ingestion of one or more cysts may cause disease, as contrasted with most bacterial illnesses where hundreds to thousands of organisms must be consumed to produce illness.

After swallowing the cyst, it reaches the intestines where it changes to its next stage and multiplies. It can also coat the lining of the intestine and prevent digestion and assimilation of foods. These parasites thrive in the small intestine and absorb nutrients from the intestinal tract. They move about with the aid of several flagella giving them a peculiar tumbling movement. With the aid of a large sucker, they attach themselves to the wall of the intestinal tract. Unattached organisms may be carried by the fecal stream to the large intestine. There, if transit time allows, the flagella are retracted and the organism develops into the infective form of the parasite and is transmitted from host to host by the fecal-oral route.

Giardia is transmitted in its cyst form through food and water contaminated by the feces of humans or animals, including dogs, cats, parakeets, beavers, muskrats, and sheep. Giardia is also found in fish, amphibians, reptiles, birds and wild animals. Hikers, backpackers and hunters pick up this parasite by dipping their canteens in a creek. Tainted stream water was so often linked to beavers that giardia infection got the nickname "beaver fever." Signs posted in wilderness areas often warn about giardia in streams. It is common in travelers, homosexuals, and children in day-care centers.

At least some strains can infect more than a single host species. Infection is highest in areas with poor sanitation and in populations unable to maintain adequate personal hygiene.

For years, it was thought that the only way to get this parasite was from drinking non-treated water, as found in mountain streams, rivers, and lakes. In the last decade, the prevalence of giardia in urban areas is rising because of inadequate water supply systems. Some infections are caused by the practice of using animal and human feces as fertilizer to grow vegetables and fruit or using contaminated water on the products. Outbreaks have been traced to food contamination by infected food handlers. The largest reported foodborne outbreak involved people who ate macaroni salad at a picnic.

The high incidence of giardia in day-care facilities may contribute to its spread from person-to-person. Infection is through contaminated food or water or through hand to mouth contact with infected articles like clothes or diapers. This is a very contagious organism with a large number of parasites being passed in a small amount of feces. One soiled diaper can harbor millions of giardia cyst. Then the children, or staff, return home passing along this parasite to other members of their family. All ages and economic groups are represented, but homosexual males, young children and young adults with impaired immune systems are more likely to acquire this parasite. Oral-anal sex is responsible for the high infection rate among male homosexuals, numbering up to 40 percent. The risks are greater if the human host already has another infection such as the yeast, *Candida albicans,* or lacks stomach acid.

Giardia organisms appear to attach themselves to the walls of the upper intestine, crippling the body's ability to absorb nutrients. Infections, such as *Entamoeba coli*, usually strike within hours, but with giardia the first rumblings probably won't appear for 7 to 14 days after exposure. It can be hard to know the source of infection when it takes this long before the first symptoms. The symptoms can vanish spontaneously, then come back repeatedly. Between times, you can feel fatigued. It can keep you miserable for as long as two weeks. After severe bouts with this organism, you may find yourself losing weight.

Symptoms, when they do occur usually begin with diarrhea that is sudden in onset and explosive in character. The stool is foul smelling, greasy in appearance and floats on water. Upper abdominal cramping is common. Large quantities of intestinal gas produce abdominal distention and belching. Nausea, vomiting, and a low-grade fever may be present. Some people begin having allergic reactions to foods. Because giardia can attach itself to the bile ducts of the liver, it can mimic gall bladder disease. If an infection with giardia is left untreated, rheumatoid and arthritic symptoms may emerge.

The acute illness generally resolves in 1–4 weeks. In children it may persist for months, leading to significant malabsorption and weight loss. In many adults, the acute phase is followed by a subacute or chronic phase. This is characterized by intermittent bouts of mushy stools, flatulence, and heartburn, and weight loss that can go on for weeks or months. After the initial bout of illness, the symptoms may decrease, but now there are only intermittent symptoms such as constipation and diarrhea. Usually the abdominal distention and foul-smelling gas persist.

Symptoms and organisms can also disappear spontaneously. This condition may be confused with a bacterial infection and the person may be subjected to unnecessary treatment. Most chronic cases are difficult to treat. Different people show various degrees of symptoms when infected with the same strain of giardia, and the symptoms may vary during the course of the disease. This is an organism that can hide in the digestive tract for years without causing any symptoms.

Giardia is one of the many microscopic organisms that can interfere with behavior, as well as physical, and mental functioning. This parasite can coat the intestinal wall, inhibiting digesting and assimilation and interfere with the absorption of nutrients such as vitamins A, B6 and B12. There may be chronic iron anemia and deficiencies of some minerals. Decreased intestinal absorption extends to oral antibiotics such as ampicillin, erythromycin, and penicillin, as well as other drugs that depend on intestinal absorption.

Some people (less than 4 percent) continue to have symptoms for more than 2 weeks after the infection is treated, because there may still be damage caused by the parasite. About 40 percent of the people diagnosed with giardia have a sugar intolerance, especially to lactose and sucrose. This intolerance to sugar and dairy can last up to six months after the infection is gone. Chronic infections lead to malabsorption and severe weight loss and are frequently hard to treat with drugs. Children may be diagnosed as having celiac disease when it is really giardia infecting them. In some immune deficient individuals, an infection with this parasite may contribute to a shortening of the life span.

Water-borne giardia came to the public's attention as far back as 1965 with several outbreaks being reported in public water supplies. The majority were surface water systems with inadequate filtration or chlorination. It seems that it is difficult to maintain appropriate concentrations of chlorine to prevent this parasite, and maybe communities should not rely upon chlorination alone to protect the public. Many small communities lack filtered water because of the cost and maintenance needed. Of 124 surface water suppliers in Massachusetts in 1985, 76 had either no filtration system or only a partial filtration system. It is even more of a risk in communities that depend on unfiltered surface water supplies.

Much of the ground water in North America has been infested with *Giardia lamblia*. This is a highly contagious organism and can be carried by virtually any species of wild animals, cats, dogs, as well as people. It can be serious among people who live in institutions and overcrowded communities and can be spread by drinking or swimming in feces-contaminated water, and from person to person, or animal to person contact.

The diagnosis of *Giardia lamblia* by standard microscopic exam can be a problem. Due to the intermittent shedding of the organism or the excretion of very low numbers of life forms, 10-50 percent of infected individuals remain undetected. It may take examining specimens at weekly intervals for over 4-5 weeks. Because giardia infections manifest symptoms that may be confused with other disease states, a misdiagnosis coupled with asymptomatic carriers, can lead to the increased spread of the infections. The distressing symptoms typically mimic bacterial food poisoning making the diagnosis even more difficult. This is why so many cases involving giardia are misdiagnosed.

Usually in acute infections the parasite can be found in the stool, but in chronic cases it may require repeated stool exams. Giardia antibodies are revealed in nearly 50 percent of patients with cysts. There are many people who have thousands of dollars done in tests and end up being treated for stress. Sometimes more invasive tests are necessary. Another technique entails swallowing a weighted gelatin capsule attached to a nylon thread. The thread is retrieved after four hours and the material on the end of the thread is examined under the microscope. Both the organisms, giardia and strongyloides, may be detected by this procedure.

Because of person-to-person spread, it is important to examine and, if necessary, treat close physical contacts of the infected person, including playmates at nursery school, household members, and sexual contacts. Provide sanitary disposal of feces and practice good personal hygiene. Many people become lax when they are at home. It is easy not to wash your hands every time the toilet is used. Children often don't want to take the time to wash their hands. Treatment should be withheld from pregnant women because of the potential toxic reaction to medication.

Hikers should avoid consuming untreated surface water, even in remote areas. All stream and mountain water should be considered infected because many animals besides humans act as hosts. Chlorination and filtering do not always eliminate the cysts. Many smaller water treatment plants are not doing a good job of ridding itself of this organism. Their outdated filters let this parasite pass right on through. All questionable water should be either boiled or treated with a product that kills giardia. It is best to cook your food and boil or filter any water used.

Flagyl (metronidazole) is normally quite effective in stopping infections. Other drugs used are paromomycin and furazolidone suspension for children. A new antigiardia agent, albendazole, is also effective against various parasitic worms including a number of nematode (roundworms) and cestode (tapeworms) species. Pregnant women should be treated only if they show significant symptoms.

LEISHMANIA TROPICA

This parasite is widespread in the tropics and subtropics. This genus of flagellate protozoa infects the blood and blood cells of its host and uses carbohydrates obtained from its host's body fluids. Several strains can infect humans. The disease recurs in epidemic form at 20 year intervals, when a new generation of non-immune children and young adults appears in the community. All species can be transmitted by sand flies.

The parasite is passed to a host when a sand fly bites a mammal. In Eurasia and South America, the domestic dog is the most common reservoir. Then the parasite is ingested by a particular type of white blood cell called a macrophage. Here is will multiply until there are so many of them that the white blood cell ruptures. Now more white blood cells rush to the area to ingest the parasites. The parasite again invades the white blood cells and multiplies there until the cell ruptures and the parasites are released and ingested by other macrophages, and this continues on and on. After being taken up with the blood by the sand fly bite, the parasite is injected into a host at the next bite.

These small, delicate, short-lived sand flies are found in animal burrows and crevices throughout the tropics and subtropics. At night, they feed on a wide range of mammals. In the eastern hemisphere, the desert gerbil serves as the reservoir host and causes infections when rural inhabitants come in close contact with the burrows of these animals. In the Mediterranean area and in India, human disease involves urban dwellers, primarily children, In this setting, the domestic dog serves as the reservoir, although sand flies may also transmit *Leishmania tropica*. It is also a disease caused by tropical and subtropical rodents. It is particularly common in areas of China, Asia Minor, Africa, and Central America.

Symptoms appear as early as two to eight weeks after the bites, but the incubation period may exceed two years. The disease exists in two major clinical forms: a skin disease and one that affects the soft organs of the gut, especially the liver and spleen. The course of the disease is determined by the species of parasite and the host's immune response.

The skin type of disease (cutaneous leishmaniasis) generally appears on the extremities or face as a small itchy, skin pimple that enlarges over time to become a swelling 1-2 centimeters in diameter that may ulcerate. Swollen lymph glands often accompanied the skin outbreak. Satellite lesions may form around the edge of the primary sore and fuse with it. Some people have several lesions. Usually the ulcers heal on their own in 3-6 months leaving a pitted, depigmented scar. Occasionally the lesions fail to heal, particularly on the ears, leading to progressive destruction of the external part of the ear. A permanent immunity follows healing.

The disease that affects the gut (visceral leishmaniasis) generally causes fever, weight loss, enlargement of the spleen and liver, and anemia. Symptoms can include high fever with chills, weakness, watery diarrhea, abdominal pain, headaches, and a chronic irritating cough. This disease can be hard to diagnose because of the varied symptoms resembling other illnesses. This form of the disease, if not properly treated, may be fatal.

Desert Storm vets may have been exposed to a new specie of leishmania. According to Army doctors, many of the cases were chemically identified as *Leishmania tropica*. However, some of the soldiers did not develop skin lesions, but manifested symptoms of the more serious form of the disease affecting the gut. The doctors admit that they know very little about this different type of *Leishmania tropica*.

Many of the soldiers returning from Desert Storm were told not to donate blood because of the possibility of contact with *Leishmania* while in the Middle East. Any soldier who was on active duty and now experiences chronic skin lesions or unexplained illness that includes fever should report to his supporting primary care medical facility for evaluation. Doctors at Walter Reed Army Hospital will provide diagnostic support to civilian physicians by doing a serum antibody test if they send the serum from their patients.

An unusual variety of the skin disease seen primarily in Ethiopia and Venezuela results in skin lesions scattered over a considerable area bearing a striking resemblance to leprosy. Since the lesions contain large numbers of organisms, this makes the diagnosis quite simple. The disease is progressive and very hard to treat. Even with drugs such as pentamidine and amphotericin B, cure is rare, but there may be a remission of the disease.

For the skin disease (cutaneous leishmaniasis or Oriental sore), a biopsy from the ulcer's edge can be done to examine or culture the organism. Drug treatment is currently available at Walter Reed hospital, where an investigational new drug protocol is available. For the localizedskin infections, sodium antimony gluconate should be given, but at half the dose and duration as with visceral leishmaniasis. Amphotericin B, cycloguanil pamoate, and pentamidine, have proven effective chemotherapeutic agents, but are generally reserved for extensive or multiple ulcerations. Advanced lesions are often hard to treat and relapse is common. Secondary bacterial infections are treated with antibiotics. Healing can take 2 to 18 months, leaving a depressed scar. Cured patients are immune to reinfection.

The gut type of disease (visceral leishmaniasis or kala-azar) is diagnosed by testing the blood, bone marrow, liver, spleen, or lymph node to examine microscopically or culture for the organism in white blood cells. This type of leishmaniasis has a mortality rate of 90 percent if untreated, but generally less than 10 percent in treated cases. Treatment with pentavalent antimonial drugs lowers this rate dramatically in many cases. Initial therapy fails in up to 30 percent of African cases and 15 percent of those that do respond eventually relapse. When this parasite is encountered in the Sudan, it is often resistant to antimony. Resistant cases are treated with the more toxic pentamidine or amphotericin B. Contact the Center for Disease Control in Atlanta for the latest drugs available for this parasite. See "Resources" for their phone number.

Prophylactic measures include the control of the sand fly vector by use of insect repellents and fine mesh screening on dwellings. Control dogs or insects where they serve as a reservoir.

There are also other species of leishmania that come from Central and South America and Mexico. They are *L. mexicana* or *L. braziliensis*. The localized lesions resemble cutaneous leishmaniasis and usually occur on the face. Untreated, the disease may persist for years with death resulting from secondary infection. The treatment of the lesions is as recommended above for visceral leishmaniasis.

PLASMODIUM FALCIPARUM

Plasmodium falciparum has been found to be a cause of malaria. There are three other kinds of *Plasmodium* besides *P. falciparum* that infect humans. They are *Plasmodium vivax*, *Plasmodium malariae*, and *Plasmodium ovale*, but they cause a less severe form of malaria. It is estimated that 40 percent of the world's population is at risk and 10 percent are at severe risk. Malaria is a major killer of children in tropical Africa, and places such as Asia and South America. It is common to find cases in adults in these areas, but now there have been reports of malaria on the east coast of this country, and an outbreak occurs yearly in San Diego, California.

These one-celled protozoans cause malaria when transmitted by an infected Anopheles mosquito. Mosquitoes that carry the malaria organism are present in almost all countries in the tropics and sub-tropics. The pathology of the disease is primarily the destruction of human red blood cells resulting in the blockage of capillaries in the gut, and impairment of the liver and other tissues. Infection may not cause any symptoms in some people, or it can be severely debilitating. Malaria can manifest as the acute malignant type or the chronic relapsing type. Acute infections may even be fatal if there is failure of several body systems.

The parasite enters a red blood cell and multiplies until it forms so many new parasites that it bursts the blood cell setting the freed parasites into the bloodstream. When this happens, the symptoms in the human host are one of chills. Now, each new parasite searches for a new red cell to inhabit and starts the process all over again. This is when the human host has a fever. Even a small number of parasites are capable of causing a high fever with shaking chills.

The life cycle of this parasite begins when a female anopheles mosquito feeds on a person who already has the malaria organism in their blood. Then they bite their next victim spreading the disease. This parasite can be introduced into the bloodstream by a transfusion of blood from an infected donor, or a common syringe used by drug addicts.

Early stages of malaria may resemble the onset of the flu. Travelers who become ill with a fever during or after travel in a malaria risk area should seek prompt medical attention and should inform their physician of their recent travel history. It should not be assumed that the traveler has the flu or some other disease without doing a laboratory test to determine if the symptoms are caused by malaria. The symptoms can develop as early as 6-8 days after being bitten by an infected mosquito or as late as several months after departure from a malaria area. Symptoms can occur every 48 or 72 hours characterized by alternating periods of chills, fever, and sweating. Sometimes there is enlargement of the spleen, headaches, muscle aches, malaise, and a chronic relapsing course of symptoms.

A malaria infection poses a serious threat to a pregnant woman and her unborn child that could include premature birth, the risk of abortion, and stillbirth. The infection may be more severe than in non-pregnant women. Pregnant women who are traveling to a malaria risk area should consult a physician and take prescription drugs to prevent this disease. It would probably be best to postpone the trip so that medication would not have to be taken.

Identification of the parasites in correctly stained blood smears is definitive. The appearance of each of the four species of malaria parasites that infect humans is sufficiently different to allow a certain diagnosis.

Any successful attack on malaria has to be made during the parasite's migration phase. Malaria can often be prevented by the use of antimalarial drugs and use of personal protection measures against mosquito bites. The risk of malaria depends on the traveler's itinerary, the duration of travel, and the place where the traveler will spend the evenings and nights. Travelers can still get malaria, despite use of prevention measures. Malaria can be treated effectively in its early stages, but delaying treatment can have serious consequences.

Since the 1960s there have been strains of *Plasmodium falciparum* in south-eastern Asia and South America showing resistance to the drug, chloroquine, making the need to develop new antimalarial drugs critical. In areas with chloroquine resistance, the drug mefloquine may be used as a malaria preventive in pregnant women. In chloroquine-sensitive areas, pregnant women can take chloroquine. Neither drug has been shown to have harmful effects on the fetus when it is used to prevent malaria. It is important to continue taking preventive medication at least for one month after leaving an endemic area.

Small amounts of antimalarial drugs are secreted in the breast milk of lactating women. The amount of drug that is transferred in breast milk does not protect the infant against malaria. All children traveling to malaria risk areas, including young infants, should take antimalarial drugs. Therefore, the recommendations for most preventive drugs are the same as for adults, but it is essential to use the correct dosage. The dosage depends on the age and/or the weight of the child. An overdose of antimalarial drugs can be fatal. Store any medication in childproof containers out of the reach of children.

Travelers on chloroquine or chloroquine/proguanil should be given a treatment dose of fansidar if at any time during their travel, they will be more than 24 hours from professional medical care. Travelers with a history of sulfonamide intolerance should not be given fansidar. If travelers develop a febrile illness and if professional medical care is not readily available within 24 hours, they should promptly take the fansidar. This self-treatment is only a temporary measure and prompt medical evaluation is imperative. For uncomplicated cases of chloroquine resistance, the recommended treatment is quinine sulfate, followed by either tetracycline or pyrimethamine-sulfadoxine. There is ongoing research to find more effective drugs in the fight against malaria. Contact the Center for Disease Control (CDC) in Atlanta for the lastest information. See "Resources" for their phone number.

Anopheles mosquitoes bite during nighttime hours, from dusk to dawn. Therefore, antimalarial drugs are only recommended for travelers who will have exposure during evening and nighttime hours in malaria risk areas. To reduce mosquito bites, travelers should remain in well-screened areas, use mosquito nets, and wear clothes that cover most of the body. Travelers should also take insect repellent with them to use on any exposed areas of the skin. The most effective compound is DEET (N,N-diethyl meta-toluamide), an ingredient in most insect repellents. However, this ingredient is known to be toxic and has caused deaths. When applying high-concentration (greater than 35 percent) of this product to the skin, particularly on children, refrain from applying repellent to portions of the hands that are likely to come in contact with the eyes and mouth.

Travelers should also purchase a flying insect-killing spray to use in living and sleeping areas during the evening and night. For greater protection clothing and bednets can be soaked in or sprayed with permethrin, an insect repellent used on clothing. If applied according to the directions, permethrin will repel insects from clothing for several weeks. Do not wear scents such as perfumes or aftershaves because they attract insects, especially mosquitoes. Some herbs and vitamins help repel fleas and mosquitoes from the body.

TOXOPLASMA GONDII

Toxoplasma gondii is common around the world and very contagious. This parasite is the cause of the disease toxoplasmosis. Approximately one-half of the human population of the United States has been infected, with the highest risk being those with AIDS, pregnant women, or women with babies. The rest of the human population is not considered a desirable host, usually resulting in infections without symptoms, and self-limiting.

Over 300 species of mammals and 20 species of birds have been identified as intermediate hosts, but this crescent-shaped protozoa can only complete its sexual cycle in the intestinal tract of felines. This includes ocelots, bobcats, cougars, and leopards, in addition to the domestic cat. Ingested parasites enter cells inside the small intestine where they mature until the cell ruptures and the parasites are released. Now, they infect other intestinal cells repeating their reproduction cycle until a cyst is formed and passed out in the feces. In the typical infection, millions of these organisms are released daily for 1–3 weeks. The cyst that is released is still immature and needs anywhere from one day to 3 weeks to mature, depending upon temperature and moisture. Once mature, the cysts may remain viable and infectious for as long as a year. These cysts are extremely small and light, and very resistant to being killed. It takes either the heat of thoroughly cooked food or very low temperatures, such as in hard frozen food, to kill this organism while in this resistant stage.

When *Toxoplasma* enters the wrong host, the organism invades cells, but not usually blood cells. The host cell eventually burst and releases more organisms that invade other cells. This will activate the host's immune system slowing down the infection. *Toxoplasma* can encase itself in a type of cyst that can survive for many years, even the lifetime of the host. It is these latent infections that can provide problems in humans.

Humans often acquire this organism from cats after direct contact with contaminated kitty litter boxes or soil where cats have placed their feces. Almost all untreated house cats are infected and passing cysts. Pregnant women should not handle the cat's litter box or even the cat. Children playing in sandboxes where cats might defecate are at high risk of contracting this organism. Breathing dust that contains infected eggs can transmit the infection.

Cysts of this organism have been found in raw milk and meat produced for human consumption and are especially common in pork and lamb, and less so in beef and chicken. It is even possible to acquire this parasite during an organ transplant. Cockroaches and flies, after being in contact with the cysts, can then infect the food you eat. An impressive amount of information links the handling and/or ingestion of raw or undercooked meat with this disease. People who often handle meat, such as cooks or butchers, are at a higher risk of infection. Another study found little difference in the number of infections between infected meat caterers and infected vegetarians.

Another way to become infected is by the congenital route. This is a congenital condition that occurs when a pregnant woman acquires toxoplasmosis for the first time, usually infected at the start of her pregnancy. This mother may not show any symptoms, but infection can take place across the placenta to the fetus. Of the infants born, about 60 percent will not show any symptoms, but the remaining 30 percent can suffer symptoms such as hydrocephalus, a condition where the abnormal accumulation of fluid in the brain causes enlargement of the skull and compression of the brain, destroying much of the brain tissue. It can also cause calcification inside the brain. Approximately nine percent will die.

The disease presents itself in three major forms: a self-limiting disease with fever and swollen lymph glands; a highly lethal infection of people with a compromised immune system; and the congenital infection of infants. Some people never show any symptoms. As with many parasitic diseases, it can take years before symptoms become obvious. The symptoms usually begin to manifest when the person's body becomes weakened or the immune system loses its effectiveness.

Some of the symptoms could include flu-like symptoms or resembling the viral infection, mononucleosis. Then it could present with chills, fever, headaches, swollen lymph glands, low blood sugar, a rash, anemia, swollen spleen, and extreme fatigue. As the disease worsens, so does the symptoms. When people are immune compromised, such as with AIDS, the parasite can affect the central nervous system, brain, lungs, eyes, and heart. An active infection can cause inflammation of the brain, paralysis, delusional behavior and headaches so bad that even painkillers do not help. A chronic phases can include symptoms such as hepatitis and swollen lymph glands. It can even look like Hodgkin's disease because of the lymph system involvement.

Approximately 1 out of every 500 pregnant women acquires acute toxoplasmosis, and in one-half of all such cases the infection spreads to the fetus. The earlier a fetal infection is acquired, the more sever it is likely to be. Overall, 20 percent of fetuses experience sever consequences. About the same amount develop a mild disease, and the remainder are without symptoms. This organism is able to cross from mother to baby causing brain and spinal cord swelling, eye infections, blindness, hydrocephalus (water on the brain), microcephaly (decreased head and brain size), brain calcifications, epileptic seizures, mental retardation, spontaneous abortion and even death.

There is a virulent form that is able to parasitize many of the same warm-blooded hosts. It is estimated that 40 percent of all cats have this parasite. It is commonly found in the brain and spinal cord. There isn't much known about this virulent specie of *Toxoplasma* or if it is infectious to people. Since *Toxoplasma gondii* is thought to infect so much of the population, there is at least a potential this other specie could be the cause of disease in those it infects.

Another similar protozoan *Sarcocystis* is contracted though eating under-cooked meat or ingesting spores. It infects the muscle tissues causing pain, swelling and degeneration. It releases a toxin called "sarcocystin" that affects the central nervous system, heart, lung, adrenal glands, liver and intestines. Use the same treatment as when treating toxoplamosis.

Toxoplasma gondii may be identified by a variety of methods including finding cysts in the feces of cats. Tests are done to the tissue or spinal fluid to isolate this parasite. Other tests such as ELISA are also available. It may be important to routinely have a blood test in those people at high risk to allow early detection and enhance the prospects of a successful outcome. Most healthy people do not require treatment unless symptoms are particularly sever and persistent, or vital organs are involved.

Prevention should be directed primarily at pregnant women and the immune compromised individuals. Hands should be carefully washed after handling uncooked meat. Cysts in meat can be destroyed by proper cooking. Since the cyst can survive normal refrigerator temperatures, it is necessary to freeze it to minus 20 °C. Pregnant women and people with impaired immune systems should never clean or change the kitty's litter pan or handle cat feces. Immune compromised and pregnant women should be treated if acute infection, or reactivation, is present.

Occasionally, it is advised to put cats outside to reduce the risk of infection with parasites such as this protozoa, *Toxoplasmosis gondii*, or the roundworm, *Toxocara cati*. An indoor cat is unlikely to pick up an infection with these organisms, since there is no ready source of contamination indoors. The litterpan is easily cleaned and most people don't dig around in the pan much. The best protection against infection is preventive treatment of the cat and regular cleaning of the litterpan. Stools should be disposed of by burning or other proper sanitation methods. Don't flush them down the toilet.

An outdoor cat, or one that goes in and out, can easily be reinfected from the soil and is very likely to defecate in places such as the garden where people tend to dig around. If you have cats, it is a good idea to wear gloves while gardening. Even if you do not have cats, what about the neighbor's cat or the ones that cruise your yard? Always properly clean vegetables grown in the garden before eating them.

Combination of sulfadiazine and pyrimethamine are available, but the last one is harmful to a fetus, and should not be used in the first trimester of pregnancy. In the United Kingdom and in France, spiramycin is the preferred drug. Another combination is the use of triple sulfonamide and folinic acid. The prognosis for AIDS patients with *Toxoplasma* is not good at present and therapy has not proven successful.

TRICHOMONAS VAGINALIS

This tiny protozoan lives in the vagina and urinary tract of females, and the prostate, seminal vesicles and urinary tract of males. Although the incidence of infection is lower in men, it is estimated that 5–15 percent of urinary tract infections are caused by this parasite, meaning that 3 million women acquire this disease each year in the United States, and that 25 percent of sexually active women are infected at any given time. Men can carry this parasite without showing any symptoms and pass it to their sexual partner, or it can persist in the male reproductive tract until symptoms manifest. Trichomonas is a sexually transmitted disease and treatment of the sexual partner(s) is necessary to prevent reinfection.

This parasite has five flagella allowing it to move actively. It also has a conspicuous supporting rod with a pointed tip that may be useful for attachment, and may also be responsible for the tissue damage produced by this parasite. *Trichomonas* eats bacteria, white blood cells, and occasionally a red blood cell in the body of its host. Although it lacks a cyst form, it can survive outside the human host for 1-2 hours on moist surfaces. In urine, semen, and water, it can live for up to 24 hours.

As mentioned earlier, this is a sexually transmitted disease. The organism can also be acquired through contact with contaminated articles. Some infections are passed through sauna benches, towels, toilet seats, and therapeutic baths. The transfer of organisms on shared washcloths may explain the high frequency of infection seen among institutionalized women. Both women and men can harbor and pass this parasite. New born female babies are occasionally found to harbor *Trichomonas vaginalis,* presumably acquiring it during passage through the birth canal.

Trichomonas can exist in the female reproductive organs. It usually infests the vagina and urethra and involves the cervix, bladder and surrounding glands. This disease is not life threatening, but manifests unpleasant symptoms. This includes a foul-smelling, white to green, cheesy, vaginal discharge that is profuse and irritating to the tissues that it touches. Other symptoms may be itching, burning, painful and frequent urination, and small vaginal lesions, as well as inflammation along the urinary tract. Sometimes the only symptoms are nonspecific urinary complaints. Although the symptoms can fluctuate in intensity, this disease can persist for weeks to months. The discharge can stop, even though the person may continue to harbor the parasite. A prolonged infection may cause damage to the reproductive and urinary tissues.

The urethra and prostate are the usual sites of infection in men. Infections are usually without symptoms because of the efficiency with which the organisms are removed from the urinary and genital tract by voided urine. When there are symptoms, they usually include recurrent pain on urination, and a scant discharge, but without any pus in the discharge.

Identification of the organism in fresh vaginal discharges, urine, or prostate secretions is definitive. This parasite is identified under a microscope by its jerky, and non-directional movements. A physical examination reveals reddened vaginal and "strawberry cervix." There is usually abundant discharge. In severe cases, there may be some bleeding from the vaginal tissues. Sometimes identification is not possible in people who do not have any symptoms and in women who have douched in the previous 24 hours. Cultures of the urinary and genital specimens may increase the number of detected cases. Unfortunately, this procedure requires several days to complete causing a delay in treatment.

During the treatment, sexual intercourse should be avoided, or use a condom if needed. This organism increases in an alkaline pH. Conditions that increase vaginal pH are progesterone that increases in the latter half of the menstrual cycle and during pregnancy, excess vaginal mucus, and overgrowth of certain bacteria such as *Streptococcus* and *Proteus.*

Metronidazole (flagyl) is extremely effective in recommended dosage, curing more than 95 percent of all infections. The vaginal tablets, dilodohydrozyquin, are available, as well as furazolidone suppositories. Simultaneous treatment of sexual partners may keep a person from being reinfected. No alcohol should be consumed when taking metronidazole and this drug should never be used during pregnancy, especially the first trimester. Sometimes the infection can be controlled with vinegar douching.

TRYPANOSOMA CRUZI
(AMERICAN TRYPANOSOMIASIS)

The American type of sleeping sickness caused by *Trypanosoma cruzi* closely resembles the African type, *Trypanosoma brucei*. It is also called Chagas' disease, affecting over 7 million people living in South and Central America. In Brazil, this form of sleeping sickness causes 30 percent of adult deaths. This disease is found in the southwestern United States suggesting that human infections are not uncommon in this area. *Trypanosoma cruzi* comprises a number of stains, each with its own distinct geographic distribution, tissue preference, and how severe of a disease they can cause.

This parasite multiplies in the gut of its host and the infective form passes out with the feces to infect the next host when bitten by an infected insect. The parasite then circulates in the host's blood invading cells where they multiply until the cell ruptures and are released to invade the bloodstream and other cells.

Transmission occurs almost exclusively in rural areas where the insect vector can find a safe harbor in animal burrows and in the cracked walls and thatch of poorly constructed buildings. The insect is a large (3 cm) winged insect that leaves it hiding place at night to feed on its sleeping hosts. It preference to bite near the eyes or lips have earned this pest the nicknames of "kissing bug" and "assassin bug." In addition to humans, a number of wild and domestic animals, including rats, cats, dogs, opossums, and armadillos, serve as reservoirs. The close association of many of these hosts with human dwellings tends to increase the incidence of disease in humans and the difficulty involved in controlling this disease. Transfusion-related infections are rapidly increasing problems in areas where this parasite is commonly found.

Most infections do not produce any symptoms. Acute infections, when they occur, are primarily in children. They begin with the appearance of a hard, non-sensitive, dull red skin lesion at the site of infection, called a chagoma, 1-3 weeks after being bitten. If the eye serves as a portal of entry, the person will present with a reddened eye, swollen lid, and enlarged lymph nodes near the ear. At the onset, there may be a sustained fever, enlargement of the liver and spleen, swelling in the extremities, or a transient skin rash. Newborns may experience acute inflammation of the brain and its membranes with symptoms persisting for week to months.

The acute phase can be followed by a chronic phase that may continue for years. The symptoms of this chronic disease usually only affects adults and includes heart or gastrointestinal problems. The symptoms can become worse until there is an enlarged esophagus and colon, as well as heart damage that includes arrhythmia, heart enlargement, and even sudden death. In 5-10 percent of people who remain untreated, they can develop severe heart involvement or brain inflammation leading to death.

The diagnosis of acute Chagas's disease rests on finding the parasite in the fresh blood or the blood may be cultured in a variety of ways. In the diagnosis of chronic disease, recovery of the organisms is not likely and diagnosis depends upon symptoms and other findings such as serum tests for antibodies.

To prevent and control this organism, there needs to be insecticides used on rural buildings where the insect is commonly found, at 2-3 month intervals. It is important to prevent transfusion-induced disease by killing the organism in all blood packs before using, or screening potential donors with blood tests. Until recently, there was not an effective drug available. At present, nifurtimox is used to treat the acute disease. It is not know if the drug really cures this disease of just suppresses the parasite. Nifurtimox does not seem to affect the organism once it has reached a chronic state. Benznidazole has proven to be effective in acute cases. For chronic cases, contact the CDC for current treatments.

Tapeworms

Tapeworms live all over the world and many different species exist. They are among the oldest parasites affecting the human race, as well as being the largest inhabitants of the intestinal tract, and the most repulsive. These long, flat, ribbon-like worms are whitish with a transparent skin-like covering. Their head (scolex) is equipped with four muscular sucking discs used to attach the worm to the

THE PARASITE MENACE / 84

intestinal wall of its host. Some species are armed with a crown of hooks. As long as the head remains in the intestinal tract, a new body can grow from it.

Next is the neck from which individual segments (proglottids) are generated one at a time to form the chain-like body. Each proglottid is a self-contained reproductive unit contain both the male and female sex organs. As the worm matures, it produces more and more segments. When the segments reach sexual maturity, they release the eggs by rupturing, disintegrating, or passing through a pore. Tapeworms do not have digestive tracts of their own, but get nourishment by absorbing partially digested substances through their skin from their human host.

Most tapeworms require an intermediate host besides humans and the worms are named accordingly, such as beef tapeworm, pork tapeworm, or fish tapeworm. Sometimes humans may serve as both the intermediate and the final host, resulting in a dangerous condition. The frequency of infection has doubled within the past ten years with the most likely reason being the popularity of eating undercooked beef and fish. Fleas are another known carrier of tapeworms, so it is possible to get them from your pets.

The adult tapeworm usually lives in the intestines of humans where they absorb nutrients, especially vitamin B12 and folic acid, as well as giving off dangerous waste products. When the adult worm rolls up in the intestines, it creates a ball under the right side of the ribs below the liver. The juvenile larva stages of certain tapeworms may burrow into various organs of the body. This larval stage is called a bladder worm or "cystircercosis." Some of them occur as a large cyst that may lodge in various organs including the heart and the brain. This cyst can be a constant source of irritation causing the body to have allergic reactions of unknown origin.

Some species have become so well adapted to living in the intestines of their human host that there may not be any symptoms. This means you can have a tapeworm and not even know that it is there. Some of the conditions and symptoms that they can cause include mineral imbalances, abnormal thyroid function, intestinal gas, blood sugar imbalances, bloating, jaundice, fluid buildup during the full moon, dizziness, unclear thinking, hunger pains, poor digestion, allergies, being sensitive to touch, weight changes, and symptoms associated with pernicious anemia.

Improvements in sanitation have really reduced the prevalence of tapeworms in the United States, but many people continue to harbor this parasite. In some parts of the world, populations take medication monthly to kill this worm. Treatment is only successful when the entire worm has been expelled. Conventional medicine considers albendazole to be the drug of choice when treating worm infections.

There are five types of tapeworms that occur in humans: the dog tapeworm (*Dipylidium caninum*), the fish tapeworm (*Diphyllobothrium latum*), the dwarf tapeworm (*Hymenolepsis nana*), the beef tapeworm (*Taenia saginata*), and the pork tapeworm (*Taenia solium*).

DIPYLIDIUM CANINUM (DOG TAPEWORM)

This tapeworm is common in dogs and cats all over the world and can be passed to humans. The louse or flea is the intermediate host, whereas humans are the final host after ingesting the louse or flea that contains the infective larva. It is very common in children because of their close association with their pets. Infants are at the highest risk when they reach the crawling age.

Children are commonly infected by kissing their dog or letting their dog lick them in the face or on the hands or fingers and then swallowing an infected flea. Petting the dog's hair and then putting unwashed hands into the mouth is another way to be infected. After the flea is swallowed, the larva is liberated. It takes about twenty days for the worm to reach maturity.

Symptoms are vague but include restlessness, itching, stomach pain, and persistent diarrhea. Children who are infected show disturbed sleep, teeth grinding, and other vague intestinal disturbances.

One way of diagnosing the dog tapeworm is by finding pumpkin-seed-like or rice grain-like particles in the stool of the child or in the undergarments. These are the egg-bearing segments (proglottids) of the tapeworm. If your dog has diarrhea off and on, sometimes drags its rear on the floor, or you find dried rice grain-like particles on the hairs of the dog's rear legs and tail, take them to the vet for deworming. Eliminate infection in your household dogs and cats. You need to thoroughly remove infected fleas from the carpets and other areas where small children may pick them up and put them in their mouth. The drugs of choice are praziquantel and niclosamide.

DIPHYLLOBOTHRIUM LATUM (FISH TAPEWORM)

Diphyllobothrium latum and other members of this genus are the broad fish tapeworms reported in humans. These are parasitic flatworms whose acute infection is called "diphyllobothriasis." Bears and humans are the final or definitive hosts for this parasite. Usually the infection involves the presence of only one worm.

The fish tapeworm is a broad, long worm, often growing to lengths of 3-7 feet at maturity and capable of attaining 30 feet. It is the longest tapeworm invading humans with as many as 4,000 segments (proglottids). The main body of the worm is virtually filled with male and female reproductive organs allowing it to produce an incredible number of eggs, often more than 1,000,000 a day. The adult attaches to the wall of the intestine with the aid of two sucking grooves located in its head (scolex).

This tapeworm is sometimes called a broad fish tapeworm, because the reproductive segments are usually broader than they are long. The adult is ivory or grayish-yellow in color and can live in humans for 20 years. The closely related worm called *Diphyllobothrium pacificum* normally matures in seals or other marine mammals and reaches only about half the length of *Diphyllobothrium latum*.

The human disease caused by the fish tapeworm was rare in the United States, although it was formerly common around the Great Lakes. It was also known as "Jewish housewife's disease" or "Scandinavian housewife's disease" because the preparers of gefilte fish or fish balls would taste these dishes before they were fully cooked. It is still common in the Baltic and Scandinavian countries and in Canada, Russia, Switzerland, Italy, Chile, Japan, and Australia. The worm was brought to North America by Scandinavian immigrants, and is now found in the midwestern states and Florida. Recently, there have been reported cases from the west coast of the United States and in Alaska.

Humans are the final host of this worm, but first it must pass through a tiny freshwater crustacean, and then to a fish. The larva that infects people, a "plerocercoid," is frequently found in the intestines of freshwater and marine fish. It is sometimes found in the flesh of freshwater fish or in fish that are migrating from salt water to fresh water for breeding.

You can be infected by eating raw, lightly cooked, under-process, pickled freshwater or certain migratory species of Alaskan salmon, perch, pike, pickerel, and American turbot. The popularity of eating raw fish dishes, such as Japanese sushi and sashimi, helps to spread this disease. Cooks who sample their fish dishes before they are properly cooked put themselves at risk of being infected. Fish tapeworms are found wherever humans, bears, and other fish-eating mammals defecate in the same lakes and streams from which the fish are obtained.

Most infected people do not produce any symptoms. During the acute stage of disease, which has its onset about 10 days after eating raw or insufficiently cooked fish, the symptoms may be similar to other tapeworm infections. This includes symptoms such as diarrhea, abdominal discomfort and pain, flatulence, vomiting, nausea, and weakness. Chronic infestations may produce some of the same symptoms or only vague discomforts including fullness in the upper abdomen, water retention, loss of weight, and malnutrition. Some people are constantly hungry because the tapeworms are eating all the food. There are times when the worm gets so large that it will cause a colon blockage.

In people who are genetically susceptible, especially those of Scandinavian heritage, a severe anemia may develop, because of this tapeworm's ability to consume most of its host's vitamin B12. Folate may be reduced as well. With the anemia that results, neurological symptoms can manifest including numbness, loss of vibration sense, and even some eye symptoms.

Microscopic identification of the yellowish-brown eggs or segments (proglottids) in the stool samples or vomit is definitive, but these eggs are difficult to distinguish from the eggs of *Nanophyetus spp.* Clinical symptoms are usually not distinctive enough for a diagnosis.

Control of this disease is accomplished by prohibiting the discharge of untreated sewage into lakes and streams. Foods are not routinely analyzed for the larva of this parasite, but microscopic inspection of thin slices of fish can be used to detect this parasite in the fish's flesh. An outbreak usually involves dishes such as sushi (a raw fish dish) made of tuna, red snapper, and salmon. It is important to cook thoroughly all salmon and freshwater fish. If you must have raw fish, freeze it to a minus 10° C for 48 hours before serving. The FDA is determining whether the freezing recommendations for raw or semi-raw seafood contaminated with roundworms, pinworms, and hookworms, will also prevent infections with the broad fish tapeworms.

Treatment is similar as described for the beef tapeworm. When anemia or neurologic symptoms are present, vitamin B12 and folate probably need to be injected. Albendazole and niclosamide are usually the drugs given. Parziquantel hymenolepsis may also be helpful.

HYMENOLEPSIS NANA (DWARF TAPEWORM)

Hymenolepsis nana is the cause of dwarf tapeworm infections. It is found in humans and is probably the one most prevalent in the southern United States. It does occur worldwide and is most frequently found in children. Infections in the same family are a common occurrence.

This is a short worm only growing 1.5 inches long at maturity with about 200 segments (proglottids). The dwarf tapeworm does not need an intermediate host, but only one mammal to host its entire life cycle. The head is small with a single ring of small hooks and four cup-shaped suckers.

The dwarf tapeworm can infect humans when the eggs are ingested from contaminated food or water, or when infected food handlers pass this parasite to others. The eggs also develop in grain beetles and many other insects, who then infect the grains that they eat. When humans eat these grains, they are also eating the parasite. Rats, mice, hamsters, and dogs can also be infected by ingesting this parasite and passing it along to humans. Most human infections result from human-to-human contact through the fecal-oral route. It is possible to be self-infected with this parasite when the eggs pass out in the stool, depending on a person's hygiene habits.

Mild infections are usually without symptoms, but if enough worms are present symptoms can include diarrhea, itching, abdominal pain, headaches, and other vague digestive complaints, especially in children. If the infection is severe the symptoms may present as body weakness, weight and appetite loss, insomnia, abdominal pain with or without diarrhea, vomiting, dizziness, allergies, nervous disturbances, and anemia. The infection may still be without symptoms even when the person has a heavy infestation.

Identification of the eggs in the feces is definitive. The eggs have two membranes enclosing an embryo with six hooklets. White blood cells may be elevated, especially the eosinophils.

One way to avoid infestation of this parasite is to prevent insect contamination of flour. It is important to control rodents. If rodents are kept as pets, they need to be dewormed. It is always important to practice good personal hygiene. The conventional drugs of choice for the treatment of dwarf tapeworm are praziquantel and niclosamide.

Humans become infected with a similar tapeworm, called *Hymenolepis diminuta,* when it infects mice, rats, and humans, after they eat cereals, grains, flour, and baking products containing infected insects (meal worms, flour beetles). Rat and louse feces are also sources of this parasite's eggs. Insects are infected when they ingest rodent feces containing worm eggs.

TAENIA SAGINATA (BEEF TAPEWORM)

The beef tapeworm is found worldwide, especially in Kenya, Ethiopia, the Middle East, Yugoslavia, and parts of Russia, and South America. It is also found in the West and Northeast parts of the United States. Infection with the beef tapeworm is common in North America, but the pork tapeworm is more prevalent in Asia, Mexico, and Latin America. *Taenia saginata* is the specific worm causing infection and usually only one worm is involved.

Taenia saginata is the second largest human tapeworm reaching a few yards long. The head (scolex) has four suckers on it, but without any hooks. The last 99 percent is just a repeating chain of half inch square reproductive segments. There can be 1,000 to 2,000 segments, known as proglottids, and they contain both male and female reproductive organs and bear the eggs. In an appropriate environment, the eggs may survive for months.

Cattle that ingest the eggs of this parasite serve as an intermediate host. Then the beef tapeworm develops into a larval stage inside the striated muscles of the cow where it becomes protected by a calcified shell. When humans ingest this parasite in raw or undercooked beef, the larval stage (called a bladder worm) turns inside out and attaches to the intestinal wall. It takes approximately 2–3 months for the worm to mature into an adult in the intestines where it thrives on a carbohydrate diet and eats the intestinal tissues for protein. Their life span can reach as long as 25 years in their host.

If the cyst phase of this parasite ends up in the central nervous system, it can result in various stages of neurologic damage including recurrent seizures or permanent disability. This condition is called "neurocysticercosis." The World Health Organization (WHO) estimates that there are 50,000 deaths worldwide every year due to this parasite. Many more survive the infection.

The ordinary freezing of raw beef does not kill the larvae unless it is for prolonged periods. Another way to be infected with this parasite is to accidentally ingest the eggs, or the more serious cyst (cysticercus), through direct or indirect fecal-oral contact with a tapeworm carrier. Cysticercosis may develop in people who do not eat beef because of contact with a carrier or by people who handle food. It is also possible to self-infect yourself.

Even with the beef tapeworm's incredible size, the adult worm living in the intestinal tract usually does not produce marked symptoms other than abdominal discomfort, chronic indigestion, or diarrhea. If there are more symptoms, they usually include abdominal cramping, nausea, nervousness, and loss of appetite. Some people complain of pain coming from the region of the stomach or of vague abdominal discomfort. Most people only realized that they are infected when they discover partial segments (proglottids) or whole pieces of the worm in their stool.

There have been reports that an infection of this parasite could produce general body weakness, weight loss, and dizziness. The worm's toxic waste can produce convulsions and seizures. If the head of this tapeworm digs in too far into the intestinal wall, these injuries can be infected with bacteria and lead to ulceration. Sometimes people have reported feeling a sensation of something crawling around in their anus. Occasionally, the proglottids may obstruct the appendix, biliary duct, or pancreatic duct.

The eggs and segments of the beef tapeworm are very hard to distinguished from those of the pork tapeworm. The proglottids may be observed on the surface of the stool or appear in the underclothing or bed sheets of the host. Passage of the proglottids may be sporadic and can be increased by excessive alcohol consumption. Another way to diagnose this worm is by the identification of the worm's head after a treatment has expelled the whole worm from the host's body. Also, segments of the worm are passed with bowel movements and may be clearly noticed.

Lab results include recovering eggs in the stool or by getting Scotch tape to adhere to the eggs around the anal opening. This is the same cellophane tape technique described for pinworm detection. Infections are detected easier with this procedure than with stool examination. If this worm has caused the more serious neurocysticercosis, then only radiographic studies, exploratory surgery, visualization of cysts in the eye, or brain scans can diagnose the condition.

In the United States, sanitary disposal of human feces has kept the transmission of the beef tapeworm at its present low rate. The parasite is readily visible and can be seen easily on inspection, if only it is done. About one percent of American cattle are infected with beef tapeworm, but only about eighty percent of the cattle are inspected. At least 25 percent of all infections are missed during routine inspection. Some parts of this country, particularly the West and Northeast, have a higher rate of infection.

In countries where sanitary facilities are inadequate, or where undercooked or raw beef is commonly eaten, the beef tapeworm is very prevalent. Thorough cooking is the most practical method of control. Salting or freezing for one week at a minus 15° C or less is also effective. It is also important to have good personal hygiene. Conventional medicine treats intestinal beef worm infections with niclosamide as the drug of choice, because it is a highly effective single-dose oral preparation. Another agent, mebendazole, may also be effective, as well as praziquantel, paromomycin, quinacrine, or niclosamide.

TAENIA SOLIUM (PORK TAPEWORM)

Taenia solium is the specific parasite causing pork tapeworm infection. It is widely distributed throughout much of the world, and is particularly common in eastern Europe, Asia, Africa, and Latin America. Transmission of the pork tapeworm no longer occurs in the United States, but travelers need to be aware of areas where it is commonly found.

The adult pork tapeworm is a shorter worm than the beef tapeworm with less than 1,000 segments (proglottids). There are usually multiple worms present rather than just one. The head has four cup-shaped suckers and a double crown of 25-30 hooks. It also has suckers on the body that attach to its host's intestinal wall. This tapeworm absorbs food through the entire length of its body. When this parasite's wastes are absorbed by its host, it produces toxic side effects. Intestinal obstruction sometimes results from the balling-up of the worm. If the head (scolex) remains attached in the gut, it will soon grow another body. The pork tapeworm can remain in the human body for 25 years or more.

The pig is usually the intermediate host of this tapeworm. When humans act as the intermediate host, the larva can penetrate the intestinal wall and invade any and all tissues of the body. Humans can also act as the final host carrying the adult worm inside their intestines and passing the eggs in the stool. When humans act as the intermediate as well as the final host, this condition is known as self-infection. Some authorities have suggested that humans may be self-infected when the mature eggs are carried backward into the stomach during vomiting. It seems more reasonable that self-infection occurs because of the transport of the eggs from the anal area to the mouth on contaminated fingers.

Once inside the human body, the egg of the pork tapeworm hatches into the larva stage and begins its life developing in the muscles. Then it spreads through the central nervous system eventually migrating throughout the body to various organs. This can cause great harm to its host when the immature larva invades the heart, eyes, liver, spine, or brain. This migration makes the pork tapeworm the most dangerous of all the tapeworms. Finally, they arrive and hook onto the upper part of the small intestines where they mature into adult worms. Inside the intestines, they can grow to 10 feet long. The relatively harmless adult tapeworm produces symptoms similar to that of the beef tapeworm.

The cyst stage, called a cysticercus, can also cause problems if it lodges somewhere inconvenient such as the brain or eye. Even if our body kills the cyst, a calcium deposit is left, so it's like carrying a small pebble around for our entire life.

Humans ingest the tiny eggs through contaminated food, water, soil, or hand to mouth contact. It is easy to become infected with the larval stage by eating raw or undercooked pork. Always Inspect the center of any pork product cooked by you or by anyone else to see if it is fully cooked. This parasite is found in fresh or smoked ham or sausage. The occurrence of pork tapeworm in humans is much less frequent than the beef tapeworm, because pork is generally well cooked. But can you really trust the cooks in the thousands of fast-food restaurants across this country?

People with adult pork tapeworm infection show symptoms similar to those discussed earlier in the section on beef tapeworms. Infection with the larval form may produce serious lesions especially in the eye or brain. Depending on the number and location of the larva in the brain, they can cause seizures and brain deterioration, often misdiagnosed as epilepsy or resembling meniogoencephalitis or a brain tumor. Nerve fiber disorders appear when the central nervous system is invaded. The death of the larva can stimulate a marked inflammatory reaction, fever, and muscle pains. When the cysts develop in the tissues of the muscles, intestines, eyes, or brain, an infected person may have muscular pains, fever, and weakness.

A diagnosis includes finding the adult worm, eggs, or segments (proglottids), in the stool. Using a Scotch tape preparation around the anus can attach the eggs or segments for testing. The microscopic eggs are thick walled and yellow-brown, but cannot be distinguished from those of the beef tapeworm. A biopsy of the brain or a brain scan can identify lesions in that location. A biopsy of lesions in other areas of the body is definitive. The central spinal fluid is often abnormal. The lab test, ELISA, is also available for diagnosing an infection with this parasite. They may be a condition called eosinophilia, where there is an abnormal amount of white blood cells called eosinophils. Fifty percent of the people diagnosed with pork tapeworm will have cysts.

Infection with the adult worm is similar to the prevention and control of the beef tapeworm. Location of the lesions will determine whether drug therapy or surgery is the treatment of choice or if an alternative can be used. Surgery may be required in some cases of brain and eye infections. The drugs of choice are praziquantel and niclosamide.

There is also a tiny roundworm called *Trichina* that infects pigs. The larvae, after burrowing into the intestinal wall, enters the blood vessels. The blood carries the larvae to the muscle fibers where these worms live and grow. Researchers have also discovered a swine virus that closely resembles the human hepatitis E virus. This may become even more of a problem if pig organs are used in human transplants. Most piglets older than 3 months are testing positive for this virus. This is just one more reason not to eat pork.

Roundworms

Roundworms are probably one of the most common parasites infecting humans, especially in meat-eating cultures. It is estimated that 200 million people worldwide are infected by roundworms because they are resistant to the various types of drug treatments. Cases in the United States have increased in the past few years. They are common in the Appalachian mountains and adjacent regions and the second most common intestinal worm in the United States.

The adult worms multiply by producing thousands of eggs each day. These eggs usually become infectious in the soil or in an intermediate host before infecting humans.

The 6-18 inch worms can be mistaken for tumors because of their habit of lumping together, or they can block the intestines. Recent research indicates the existence of worms as part of the cause of many more health problems than was previous believed. Even some cases of cancer are thought to be caused by the infestation of worms.

If the infection is mild, there are not any symptoms, and the human host can accommodate these parasites without even knowing it. If the worm reproduces in great numbers and creates organ obstruction, then symptoms become obvious. In heavy roundworm infections, it is common to see nutritional deficiencies and even appendicitis, especially in children. A heavy infestation usually means that some underlying cause in the host provided a suitable habitat for the worms. It could mean that the host had so many repeated exposures to the parasite that infection was bound to happen. Given these circumstances, the removal of the worm(s) will not make the person healthy or prevent reinfection.

In trying to eliminate intestinal worms or parasites the use of poisons or drugs are the conventional approach, but may be debilitating to the patient. Since the reproduction of these worms requires that a portion of its life cycle be outside the human body, continuing infection almost always implies the practice of improper hygiene. Prevention and treatment greatly depend on the proper washing of foods, disposal of waste matter, and good hygiene. If a patient has worms, boil all their underwear and bedding to help prevent reinfection. It is also important to consider the living conditions, diet and nutritional status, general state of health, and the integrity of the stomach and bowels of anyone at risk or infected with roundworms. A child's poor hygiene can infect other family members, play mates, and other people that come in contact with the child. An infected child's close associates should also be examined.

ANCYLOSTOMA CANINUM (HOOKWORM)

This is a type of hookworm that can infect humans, but usually is found in man's best friend, the dog. Upon contact with soil contaminated with dog or other animal feces, the larva, which lives in the soil, burrows into the skin of the human. Since it is unable to penetrate deep into the tissues, the worm just travels around the skin causing a disease called "creeping eruption." The skin itches, but after a few months the worm dies. Refer to other hookworms below for drug treatment.

ANISAKIS SIMPLEX (FISH ROUNDWORM)

Fertilized eggs from the female parasite pass out of the host with the feces. In sea water, the eggs developing into larvae that hatch in sea water. Minute crustaceans related to shrimp, and other small invertebrates, become infected. The larvae grow in these animals and become infective for the next host, a fish or something such as a squid. The larvae may penetrate through the digestive tract into the muscle of the second host, Some evidence exists that the larvae move from the gut to the flesh if the fish is not gutted promptly after catching.

The life cycles of all the other *Anisakis* species implicated in human infections are similar. These parasites are known to occur frequently in the flesh of cod, haddock, fluke, pacific salmon, herring, flounder, and monkfish. It has been found in the stomachs of whales and dolphins. These worms produce a substance that causes an immune reaction from the host's body causing white blood cells, including eosinophils, to rush to the area in defense. One worm is all it takes to infect a person, but they rarely reach full maturity in humans and are usually eliminated spontaneously from the digestive tract within 3 weeks of initial infection. Worms that penetrated other tissues are eventually removed by the host's white blood cells.

To get *Anisakis,* all you need to do is eat raw or undercooked seafood containing the larvae. This means eating pickled or salted marine fish or squid. These roundworms have been implicated in human infections in places such as northern Europe and Japan. Japan has the greatest number of reported cases because of the large volume of raw fish consumed there.

A recent letter to the editor of the *New England Journal of Medicine* stated that approximately 50 cases of infection caused by *Anisakis* have been documented in the United States, to date. Three cases in the San Francisco Bay area involved ingestion of sushi or undercooked fish. This is one parasite that is going to be seen more often with the increasing popularity of sushi and sashimi in restaurants.

The letter also points out that an infection with this organism is easily misdiagnosed as some other illness such as acute appendicitis, Crohn's disease, gastric ulcer, or gastrointestinal cancer. Some chronic cases last longer than a year. In North America, this parasite causes the affected individual to feel a tingling or tickling sensation in the throat prior to coughing up and then having to manually extracting a worm or it will be swallowed and end up in the intestines. In more severe cases there is acute abdominal pain appearing like acute appendicitis, accompanied by a nauseous feeling. Symptoms occur from as little as an hour to about 2 weeks after the consumption of raw or undercooked seafood. Other symptoms include fever and diarrhea. The symptoms apparently can persist after the worm dies since some lesions are found upon surgical removal that contain only remnants of the worm. If the parasite does perforate the intestinal wall, it can cause peritonitis, leading to death.

Candling or examining fish on a light table is used by commercial processors to reduce the number of *Anisakis* in certain white-flesh fish that are known to be infected frequently. This method is not totally effective or even adequate to remove the majority of worms from these fish.

In cases where a person vomits or coughs up the worm, the diagnosed can be made by identifying the worm. Other cases may require more sophisticated technology. One way is to use a fiber optic device that allows the attending physician to examine the inside of the stomach and the first part of the small intestine. These devices are equipped with a mechanical forceps that can be used to remove the worm.

Conventional treatment includes resection of the damaged wall, antibiotic therapy for secondary infections, and in some cases removing the larva form the stomach with a fiberscope. In severe cases the worm needs to be surgically removed. In order to prevent and control this parasite it is best to cook or freeze fish, as well as gut and salt fish immediately after catching. The FDA recommends that all fish and shellfish intended for raw (or semiraw fish such as marinated or partly cooked) consumption be blast frozen for 15 hours, or be regularly frozen to a minus 10° F, or below, for 7 days.

ASCARIS LUMBRICOIDES
(GIANT INTESTINAL ROUNDWORM)

Twenty-five percent of the world's population, including 4 million Americans, are infected with roundworms. The southern part of this country and the Appalachian region has the highest infestation rate.

It is often found in moist climates where soil pollution is common. Whether you live in the country or in urban America, you are equally prone to infection by this parasite.

Ascaris is the largest of the round worms, reaching 6-16 inches in length as thick as a pencil, and weighing the most. It is pink with bright red speed stripes. It doesn't eat us or cause a bad reaction to its presence, but because of it size it is capable of causing all sorts of trouble. If we try to kill it with worming medication, it has the ability to move up the body causing vomiting of giant worms. If it moves in the other direction, we can find some unpleasant things in the toilet.

Once the eggs are ingested and become larvae in the small intestine, they can penetrate the intestinal lining and enter the bloodstream and the lymphatic system on their way to the liver. As *Ascaris* matures, it moves from the right side of the heart to the lungs. During the last phase of migration the adult ends up back in the small intestine where it breeds. The female grows as long as a foot and begins production of enormous numbers of eggs (27 million in her lifetime) which are excreted in the feces. The adult worm can live for more than a year.

The eggs live outside of the host's body in temperatures ranging anywhere from 59.9° to 100.4° F. This is why *Ascaris* lives in warm areas of the world. The eggs become infective after 2-3 weeks in the soil, where they can survive up to seven years in the typical urban yard.

Food coming from south of the border carries the biggest risk. The mature eggs are most often spread because food, and people's fingers, have been contaminated with human fecal matter, particularly in areas of the world where night soil (human feces) is used for fertilizer. This could include unwashed fresh fruits or vegetables. Children are commonly infected by eating dirt or placing soiled fingers or toys in their mouths. Even airborne dust can carry *Ascaris* eggs into nasal passages and mouths.

These worms compete for food and inhibit absorption of proteins, fats, and carbohydrates. Yet, many people do not have any obvious symptoms with the initial infection. Symptoms in adults can be vague, but there can be abdominal pain, swelling of the lips, allergic reactions, insomnia, anorexia, and weight loss. The person may have a full, pale upper lip, and white lines around the mouth.

It is possible to have an allergic reaction to the toxins this parasite produces. The resulting symptoms can include asthma, insomnia, eye pain, and a skin rash. As the larvae migrate, they can cause inflammation in the spleen, liver, lymph nodes and brain. Lung infections may be accompanied by a fever, coughing, and difficulty breathing. If there are enough adult worms in the intestinal tract, mechanical blockage may be possible. Adult worms can penetrate the intestinal wall or appendix causing local hemorrhage and appendicitis.

The common symptom picture in children may also include convulsions or spasms, nervousness, irritability, twitching in various parts of the body, itching or irritation of the nose or the anus, oral pallor, poor or ravenous appetites, restlessness at night, and dry cough or wheezing. Children infected with *Ascaris* can have a lactose tolerance and impaired absorption of vitamin A. They also frequently pick their nose.

The diagnosis is usually made by finding the eggs in the feces. Because of the extreme productivity of the female worm, it generally makes this task easy. When this parasite is infecting the lungs, then a diagnosis is made by finding the larva in the sputum. There may white blood cells, called eosinophils, in the sputum as well as adult worms. Infection by immature or only male worms can be detected only radiologically. It is common to find other intestinal parasites in association with *Ascaris*.

When considering a treatment plan, it is important to know that a mild *Ascaris* infection is common in childhood. If the child is healthy and there are not any symptoms, this parasite is not considered a serious problem requiring treatment. If the community is heavily infested, then there needs to be community wide control of this parasite with mass therapy given at 6 month intervals. Ultimately, it takes adequate sanitation facilities to control this worm. Pyrantel pamoate and mebendazole are highly effective with the latter being preferred. Other drugs are piperazine citrate and albendazole. Most people respond to just one dose. If the infections are concurrent with *Giardia lamblia* and *Entamoeba histolytica*, treat for *Ascaris* first to avoid provoking worm migration, intestinal perforation, or causing the worms to knot up.

DIROFILARIA IMMITIS (DOG HEARTWORM)

This parasite is found worldwide. In the United States, the dog heartworm is most commonly found in the Mississippi River Valley and the Atlantic and Gulf Coast. This is a tiny blood and tissue-dwelling roundworm common in dogs and other mammals. It is transmitted through the bite of a mosquito. The tiny juveniles live in the gut of a mosquito and passed from host to host through its bite.

The mature worm does not usually live in humans, but the larvae can. In humans it lives in the heart, blood vessels and lungs causing a cough and chest pain. In severe cases, it can cause blockages of the blood vessels, damaging various organs. The dog heartworm is becoming increasingly common. The drug, diethylcarbamazine, has possibilities since it kills other kinds of microfilariae in the blood.

ENTEROBIUS VERNICULARIS (PINWORM)

Over 200 million people worldwide are thought to be infested by pinworms with 30 to 40 million living in this country. This worm is found in both warm and cold climates and no socioeconomic group is immune to infection. It is commonly found in crowded institutions such as day-care centers, schools, mental hospitals, and orphanages.

It is the most common worm infection in this country, and is most prevalent in children. Also called "seat" or "thread" worms, these 1/4 inch mobile worms resemble threads. They are tiny, 2-13 millimeters, and ivory or pearly-white in color. Eighty percent of the children between 2 and 10 years of age contract pinworms at some time.

Adult worms inhabit the cecum and other portions of the large and small intestines. Female worms crawl down the intestines and pass out of the anus to lay their eggs around the anal region at night. Occasionally, they can be found on the first stool in the morning. One female pinworm can deposit over 15,000 eggs that become infective immediately or within a few hours.

This common occurring worm is acquired through contaminated food, water, and house dust, as well as human-to-human contact. The crawling of the female worm on the skin around the anal area often produces intense itching causing a person to scratch there, getting the eggs on the hands. Without washing, the hands touch the mouth. Now the eggs are swallowed and hatch in the lower colon where the worms mate, and the cycle continues.

The eggs are usually found on the infected person's pajamas and bed linen. Children can easily infect the entire family through the bathtub, toilet seat, and bedclothes. The eggs are easily transported by air currents making it common to find them in every room of the house on sheets, clothes, walls and carpets. They can stay viable for weeks. Infections and reinfections continue by wearing clothes or sleeping in the bed of an infected person, as well as handling infected pets. It can be passed from an infected person that handles the food in the household. If one person in the family has pinworms, it is common to find others infected as well. This is a very contagious parasite.

Complications are much more common in women than in men. This stems from the fact that the female worm, after depositing her eggs, loses her way while trying to return to the colon. She enters the vagina instead, traveling up to the uterus and fallopian tubes.

Itching around the anal or vaginal areas are the most common pinworm symptoms. Suspect a pinworm infection if your child shows night time itching in these areas. Symptoms also include poor appetite, teeth grinding, hyperactivity, nervousness, irritability, insomnia, bed wetting, stomach aches, nausea and vomiting. There have been cases of epilepsy and vision problems caused by pinworm infections. Heavy infestations of pinworms can cause mental depression and anorexia. Sometimes the anal area becomes infected with bacteria because of the constant scratching. Pinworms are often found within the appendix and have been associated with acute and chronic inflammation.

Egg are seldom found in the feces. A parent needs to inspect the child's rectal area at night when the child is sleeping for evidence of the parasite. One way is to perform a Scotch tape test. The first thing in the morning pat the sticky side of the Scotch tape around the child's anal opening. Fold the tape together with the smooth side out, and send or bring the tape to your physician, or the laboratory, to be tested.

To control and prevent infection and re-infection from pinworms, bathe daily, but use one washcloth and towel for the face and hands, and another for the rest of the body. Don't reuse the towels before washing them. It is important to scrub hands after bathroom use and before eating. Keep toothbrushes in containers so they will not be contaminated. If there is someone infected in the household, they need to wear close-fitting underpants at all times, even when sleeping, and not share the bed with others. Bed linens and personal clothing must be wash daily. Scrub toilet seats, and clean and vacuum daily to remove eggs. Keep all rooms well aired out. Superheat the house or room to 95° F for one day. If you do this, be sure that all pets and family members are out of the house.

Conventional medicine uses pyrantel pamoate and mebendazole for treatment. Also used are albendazole and piperazine. It may be necessary to treat all members of a family simultaneously. In severe infections, re-treatment after 2 weeks is recommended, because reinfection is extremely common.

EUSTRONGYLIDES SPP. (FISH ROUNDWORM)

These large, bright red roundworms, 25-150 millimeters long and 2 millimeters in diameter can be seen without magnification in the flesh of fish. They occur in freshwater, brackish water, and marine fish and are very active after the fish's death. The larvae normally mature in wading birds such as herons, egrets, and flamingos, especially after they eat minnows.

One live larva is all it takes to cause an infection in humans. Fortunately, the disease is extremely rare; only five cases reported in the United States. If the larvae are consumed in undercooked or raw fish, they can attach to the wall of the digestive tract. One case was reported from the consumption of sashimi, a raw fish dish.

In the cases where clinical symptoms have been reported, the penetration of the parasite into the gut wall was accompanied by severe pain. The worm can perforate the gut wall and probably other organs. Removal by surgical resection or fiber optic devices with forceps is possible if the worm penetrates accessible areas of the gut. The worm can be identified after its removal. Complications could include blood poison from the amount of bacteria in the blood as a result of the perforated digestive tract. In one case, there was no clinical data and in another, the patient was treated medically and recovered in 4 days.

NECATOR AMERICANUS/ANCYLOSTOMA DUODENALE (HOOKWORM)

Necator americanus is found in the tropical areas of Asia, Africa, and America, as well as the southern United States, where it was introduced with the African slave trade. *Ancylostoma duodenale* is seen in the Mediterranean basin, the Middle East, northern India, China, and Japan. It has been estimated that together these two worms extract over seven million liters of blood each day form 700 million individuals scattered around the world. *Necator americanus* means "American murderer." Not all infections cause disease. It usually takes more than 25 adult worms to cause disease and the people who are the most likely to be infected have poor nutrition.

Adult hookworms are small, cylindrical, grayish-white with a head that is often curved in a direction opposite that of the body. This is what gives them the hooked appearance. Both species infect humans, but one possesses four sharp toothlike structures, whereas the other has cutting plates. These are the only worms that have teeth. The larvae enter the human body through the skin, travel to the lungs, up the respiratory tract until they are swallowed and end up in the small intestines. They will grip onto the intestinal wall often penetrating it until they reach a small blood vessel.

Once the hookworms find a blood vessel, they will inject an anti-coagulant into the blood to prevent the blood from clotting. In this way, the hookworm is insured of a good supply of blood. Because hookworms suck blood, they are often colored red. Hookworms also bite and suck on the intestinal wall causing bleeding and tissue death. In severe infections, so much blood is lost as to cause an iron deficiency. They can live in humans for 15 years extracting .2 to .3 ml daily, resulting in an enormous blood loss over time. The females can each release 10,000 to 20,000 eggs daily.

You can get hookworms from walking barefoot on infected warm, moist soil or by using your bare hands to garden. The eggs are usually deposited on shady, well-drained soil. The larvae develop under conditions of abundant rainfall and high temperatures. When there is direct contact with unprotected human skin, infection by the larvae can take place. Infections become particularly intense in closed, densely populated communities, such as tea and coffee plantations. Part of the life cycle of the hookworm is surviving as a free living worm outside the body. This means that they can live in water or soil. This is where humans commonly pick up the infection, but it is also through eating fruits, vegetables or drinking water contaminated with the larva stage of the worm.

Where the worm first penetrates the skin, it causes a condition known as "ground itch." This can be accompanied by intense itching and burning, swelling and redness. As the worm migrates, it produces symptoms of hemorrhaging, dry cough, and a sore throat. As the adults actively feed the results are iron deficiency anemia, intermittent abdominal pain, loss of appetite, and on occasion you see a craving to eat soil. Heavy infection creates an environment for bacterial infections, a more severe anemia, protein deficiency, dry skin and hair, edema, distended abdomen especially in children, stunted growth, delayed puberty, and mental dullness. In severe cases with much blood loss, the person may suffer cardiac insufficiency and even death.

Chronic infections may involve a worsening of the iron anemia, heartburn, flatulence, hunger pains, abdominal tenderness, irritability, alternating diarrhea and constipation, dry skin, and even blurred vision. There are some types of hookworms that don't usually infect humans. When they enter the wrong host, the juvenile hookworms migrate under the skin causing considerable skin damage before they are attacked by a person's immune system.

The identification of eggs in fecal smears is definitive. Prevention requires improved sanitation. Treatment includes improved nutrition especially increased protein and specific focus on the anemia. Iron therapy may be indicated. The drugs of choice are mebendazole, pyratel pamoate, and albendazole.

STRONGYLOIDES STERCORALIS (THREADWORM)

This parasite, commonly called a threadworm, is found in Southeast Asia, the Middle East, South America, and in people returning from these areas. Infections can be acquired in the southern part of the United States, since this is part of *Strongyloides'* range. The life cycle and pathology of this roundworm is similar to the hookworm, except the eggs hatch into larvae inside the intestine before passing in the feces. The life cycle begins by a worm larva burrowing into the skin of a human host. It them passes through the circulatory system and ends up eventually in the lungs, up the trachea and swallowed, maturing in the intestines where eventually they will re-infect the original host. Strongyloides is unique in that the mature adult worm can reproduce entirely in the human host or grow into a free-living worm in the soil.

The infection is transmitted when the larvae penetrate the human skin or hair follicles. They usually attack and enter between the toes or at the bottom of the foot reaching maturity in the intestines. When the larvae invade the intestinal wall and the lungs, a condition known as disseminated strongyloides develops; this condition can be fatal. *Strongyloides* can be transmitted by dog, cat, fox, as well as pigs, rodents, and horses. Whether humans will be infected, or not, depend on the organism strain.

This parasite is mostly harmless if there is a functioning immune system. Otherwise, this tiny roundworm is capable of infecting every organ and part of the body. Even if someone is a carrier, they can develop serious illness years after the initial infection if the immune system is compromised such as in AIDS, chronic fatigue syndrome, or if the person suffers from malnutrition. Steroid therapy puts people at a high risk for infection.

People infected with Strongloides do not usually have "ground itch" as with hookworm infection. They do have the pulmonary disease seen in both *Ascaris* and hookworm infection. Mild infections may be without symptoms. More severe infections may be marked by abdominal pain and bloating, nausea, vomiting, alternating diarrhea and constipation, and greasy stools. The liver and pancreas ducts, the entire small bowel, colon, heart, lungs, and central nervous system may all be involved in malabsorption.

With a heavy worm load, the person may complain of heartburn and tenderness often aggravated by the intake of food. A peptic ulcer-like pain associated with an elevated eosinophil count on a blood test suggests a diagnosis of Strongyloides infection. Chronic severe infections may produce anemia, weight loss, chronic dysentery, and a low-grade fever. Reinfection can lead to a chronic disease state that may last for up to 30 years.

Laboratory results include finding a high count of the white blood cells called eosinophils. Eggs are rarely found in the stool except after a violent purge or in cases of diarrhea. The presence of the infective form of larvae in fresh feces is more common. The number of larvae passed in the stool varies from day to day, often requiring several specimens before the diagnosis of Strongyloides can be made. If the lung system is involved, the sputum should be examined for larvae. If the feces are cultivated for 48 hours, larvae and free-living adults may be found. It is important to differentiate between the different types of hookworms.

Anyone living or visiting areas where this parasite is common, or if they are taking immune-suppressive drugs, should be tested with at least three stool specimens to rule out this parasite and avoid the risk of being infected. Medical personnel caring for patients with an infection of this parasite should wear protection from the stool, saliva, vomit, and body fluids, because they can contain the infectious larvae. The drugs of choice are thiabendazole, mebendazole, cambendazole, albendazole, and ivermectin. Check stools after treatment to be sure the parasite is gone.

TOXOCARA CANIS & CATI (DOG & CAT ROUNDWORMS)

These roundworms cause visceral larva migrans, found mainly in children. The eggs of these parasites get into the food and water and are ingested. Humans are not the best host for the mature worm, but it is the larvae that cause disease in humans. When the larvae hatch, they travel to various parts of the body such as the lungs, liver, brain, or eye.

Toxocara canis is found in the intestine of dogs whereas *Toxocara cati* is the name of the parasite found in cats. This is a major concern because they are transmissible to people. Children are especially at risk because of their playing and unsanitary habits around pets. Most puppies and kittens are infected. There should be care taken when handling and cleaning up around unwormed animals.

The eggs develop in the intestinal tract where they mature and burrow into the circulatory or lymph system and eventually reach the liver and then the lungs. In animals these larvae complete their life cycle by passing from the lungs into the trachea, being coughed up and reswallowed where they can mature in the intestines. The life cycle cannot be completed in humans. Instead, the worm wanders through the body causing damage. The liver, lungs, heart, skeletal muscle, brain, and eyes are involved most frequently.

Since people get infected by somehow ingesting dirt infected with the animal's feces, it is important to eliminate the problem with proper hygiene and deworming of the dog or cat. A dog with a mild roundworm infection can pass 10,000 eggs in every gram of stool. If you add this to the other 80 million dogs in America, you have many potential worm infections. Some surveys have detected these eggs in up to 30 percent of the public parks, urban backyards, and children's sandboxes.

The severity of infection is related to the number and location of the worms and the degree of sensitivity the host has to the larvae. The symptoms could include a fever, joint and muscle pains, vomiting, liver and/or lung problems, a rash, or even convulsions. The liver can enlarge and abdominal pain can occur, as well as pneumonia. *Toxocara* has been known to lodge in the eye causing inflammation and blindness.

Stool examination is not helpful since this parasite seldom reaches adulthood in humans. It usually takes something such as a liver biopsy to confirm a diagnosis of this worm. A less invasive test is called ELISA that may detect elevated antibodies in the body by the use of a blood test. Usually a diagnosis is made on the symptoms and if there is elevated eosinophils, a type of white blood cell, in the blood. Prevention requires control of dog and cat feces and repeated worming of household pets. Worming needs to begin when the puppies are 2-3 weeks of age and the kittens are about 6 week old, and repeated every 3 months during the first year of life and twice a year thereafter. Conventional treatment may include corticosteroid treatment in serious pulmonary, heart, or central nervous system involvement. Some of the more common worm medications are not that effective. The usual ones used are diethylcarbamazine, thiabendazole, and mebendazole.

TRICHINELLA SPIRALIS (PORK ROUNDWORM)

This roundworm infection can masquerade as many illnesses. *Trichinella spiralis* is the tiny worm that causes trichinosis. It is commonly found in this country, but usually without symptoms or only mild ones, since symptoms are related to the severity of the infection. This small spiral-shaped roundworm is not transmitted through soil contaminated by feces like other worms in this group. Instead, it becomes enclosed in a cyst inside the muscles of mammals, especially pigs.

If the meat that is eaten is not cooked thoroughly, the cysts are dissolved by the host's digestive juices, releasing the worm in the intestinal area where it matures, mates, and releases a huge number of young worms. These juveniles now burrow out of the intestines causing symptoms. They can migrate into blood vessels and wander all over the body, eventually ending up in the muscle fibers where they are happy to live and grow. They can also burrow themselves into various organs such as the larynx, abdomen, chest, diaphragm, jaws and upper arms. They do this with a spear-like burrowing tip on the anterior part of their body. Here they calcify, causing severe muscle soreness and fever. The adult worm is not commonly seen. Meat from pigs, bears, and seals is the principal source of infection. Humans usually become infected through eating the cyst present in the muscle of pigs made into pork products.

As this worm goes through its various stages, so many different symptoms can manifest that it is hard to believe that they are caused by just one parasite. It can look like food poisoning. It can cause acute diarrhea, nausea, vomiting, fever, colic, and symptoms of a low-grade infection, when the worms penetrate the first part of the small intestine. After *Trichinella* migrates to muscle tissue in about 2–4 weeks, there will be severe muscle pain. When the larvae finally encyst themselves in the muscle fiber, there can be extreme dehydration and toxic swelling of the lip, face, or eyelids, as well as difficulty breathing. Worms that don't encyst and stay in the larva stage can penetrate other organs and tissues. When the infection becomes this severe there are enlarged lymph glands, and swelling of the brain, resulting in damage. Other symptoms include exhaustion and lung embolism. The disease could manifest as pneumonia, pleurisy, kidney disease, and cardiac failure. The waste products that *Trichinella* produces are toxic, adding to the symptoms.

Identification of living, coiled larvae within biopsy material is definitive. However, diagnosis may also be based upon other tests such as ELISA that is capable of detecting specific antibody formation during the first week of illness. The blood test usually indicates that white blood cells, called an eosinophils, are elevated.

Be especially careful when eating pork. Even a small taste of undercooked sausage can lead to a huge infection. Cooking pork in a microwave does not assure that the cysts have been killed. Pork should be cooked until there is absolutely no pink left in the meat. The drug, mebendazole, may shorten the course of the infection Thiabendazole is also highly effective.

TRICHOSTRONGYLUS (HERBIVORE ROUNDWORM)

Throughout the world this parasite commonly infects the digestive tract of herbivore animals. Humans are usually an accidental host. Light infections usually do not cause any symptoms, but severe infections may produce a mild anemia, emaciation, dry skin, and symptoms of intestinal hemorrhage. It can be hard to differentiate between an infection caused by *Trichostrongylus,* or if it is coming from those of hookworms, or a *Strongyloides* species. Identification depends on the detection of eggs or the recovery of adult worms in the stool. The drugs of choice are pyrantel pamoate, mebendazole, or albendazole.

TRICHURIS TRICHIURA (WHIPWORM)

These common parasites are found throughout the world, infecting approximately one billion people, especially children. The eggs develop in the small intestine where they can later travel into the large intestine to mature. These 30–50 millimeter whip-shaped worms inject a digestive fluid that converts the colon tissue into a liquid that the worms can consume.

People returning from areas of poor sanitation in the warmer, humid climates, such as the Tropics, find themselves infested with whipworms. Most of these worms live in the cecum, the large pouch forming the beginning of the large intestine. If there is a heavy infestation, it is possible to find them throughout the entire large intestine. Humans become infected when they ingest eggs from contaminated soil or water that gets on vegetables and fruits. One female can lay 3,000 to 7,000 eggs a day.

Light infections may not cause any symptoms. If the infection becomes worse, there may be abdominal pain, localized tenderness, nausea, vomiting, constipation, gas, a slight fever, and headaches. Infections can become so severe that the symptoms are characterized by frequent bloody diarrhea, abdominal pain and tenderness, weight loss, anemia, and possible rectal prolapse. There have been cases of whipworm infection causing fatalities.

There are usually so many eggs in a sample of feces that a diagnosis of whipworm infection is easily made. If there are not any symptoms, infections are not usually treated. Mebendazole is the drug of choice, although the cure rate is only 60–70 percent. Some success is found with albendazole. Prevention consists of improving hygiene and sanitation.

Flukes

The most common form of parasite found in humans worldwide is likely to be a fluke, also called a trematode. Once they invade humans, flukes are very difficult to get rid of and very destructive. Typically, the adult fluke lives for decades within human tissues and blood systems, while resisting attacks from the immune system. There are many species of flukes, but they are usually put into four groups: liver, intestinal, lung, and blood flukes. I have also included the fish-flu fluke. The diseases they cause are thought to be uncommon in the United States at this time, but people returning from Asia or the Tropics are often infected.

Flukes are generally flat with an oval or leaf-like shape and grow to 3.5 inches in length. They possess two suckers, one surrounds the mouth cavity and the other is located on the body. They use these suckers for attachment and inchworm-like movement. Their reproductive system varies and divides the fluke into two categories: one form contains both the male and female sex organs, while the other form has separate sexes. If the larvae contain both sexes, they form a cyst in or upon an aquatic plant or animal, where they undergo transformation to become infective. Their cycle is completed when the second intermediate host (vegetation, fish, or shell fish) is eaten by a human. Flukes are parasitic during most of their life cycle no matter what form they assume.

Flukes can end up in various organs releasing many eggs that eventually work their way into either the digestive or urinary tract. Before the eggs pass out of the body, they can cause extensive inflammation and damage because each egg has tiny spines on the outside of them. They commonly infect the intestines, but it is possible to find them in the lungs, heart, brain, liver, and blood vessels. The worms also release toxic by-products that can damage the host's tissues.

CLONORCHIS SINENSIS (LIVER FLUKE)

Liver flukes are common in the Far East, particularly in Korea, Japan, Taiwan, the Red River Valley of Vietnam, the southern Chinese province of Kwantung, and Hong Kong. Immigrants from these areas have an infection rate of anywhere from 15 to 23 percent. In some villages in southern China, the entire adult population is infected. People who live or visit areas where this parasite is prevalent are at high risk of infection.

Clonorchis sinensis, the Chinese liver fluke, is a small, slender, flat worm that grows up to 20 millimeters long. There is a large sucker in the mouth, as well one on the body. The body also contains both the male and female sexual organs. The liver fluke can survive 30 years in a human by feasting on the rich secretions. About 2,000 tiny, light yellowish-brown eggs are released daily and find their way down the bile duct and into the fecal stream. When the eggs reach fresh water, they are eaten by a snail host allowing the flukes to continue their life cycle. Then they are passed from the snail to penetrate the tissues of freshwater fish. If the infected fish is eaten by a fish-eating mammal, such as humans, the larvae are released in the small intestines, move to the bile duct and capillaries of the gallbladder or liver, and mature to adulthood over the next 30 days.

Snails, carp, and many species of fish are known to be intermediate hosts. Another way to spread this parasite is the practice of fertilizing commercial fish ponds with human feces (night soil). When you eat raw, dried, salted, pickled, frozen, or undercooked fish, you are putting yourself at risk of acquiring this or some other parasite. A shipment of food products carrying this fluke travels long distances from its original source.

Infection with the liver fluke may not cause any obvious symptoms if the infection is light, but severe infections may be characterized by an enlarged and tender liver and jaundice, suggesting hepatitis. If you have these symptoms along with a history of travel to areas where these parasites live, there is certainly a possibility of being infected with the liver fluke. Some people complain of feeling poisoned and having pain in the right side of the body, possibly due to the many holes made throughout the liver by the worm.

Other symptoms could include edema, diarrhea, a fast heart beat, palpitation, vertigo, inflammation, chills, fever, and mental depression. The disease is rarely fatal in itself, but the host may be at a higher risk of getting other infections as a result of lowered resistance. Numerous reinfections may produce a worm load of 500 to 1,000 worms, resulting in the formation of bile stones. People with severe, long-standing infections can have cancers develop. Dead worms may obstruct the common bile duct and create an environment for bacterial infection. Occasionally, adult worms are found in the pancreatic ducts, where they can produce obstruction and acute pancreatitis.

The eggs are identified on microscopic examination in stool samples or in bile. In mild infections, it may take repeated examinations before the parasite is found. Since most people are without symptoms, it is important to also rule out other causes of illness. Look for elevated white blood cells, especially eosinophils, on a blood test, as well as elevated alkaline phosphatase levels. The liver could be abnormal on ultrasonographic scans. There are other tests that could reveal enlargement of the bile ducts in the liver and gallbladder.

To prevent infection, eat only cooked fresh-water fish, especially in areas where these parasites live. Prevent contamination of fish ponds by human feces and from other infected meat eaters. Where there have been improvements in the disposal of human waste, there have also been decreases in the liver fluke. Unfortunately, the extremely long life span of these worms keeps them reproducing in the environment. The drug, praziquantel, may be an effective therapeutic agent.

FASCIOLOPSIS BUSKI (INTESTINAL FLUKE)

The adult fluke lives in the small intestine where it can cause ulcerations. The female produces eggs that hatch in the intestinal tract producing larvae that sprout tails and can swim in the fluid. After a short period, the tails drop off so that the flukes can encircle themselves with a protective cocoon, forming the next stage. According to Dr. Hulda Clark, Ph.D., N.D., this stage of development produces a thick shell that propyl alcohol and other solvents in our body fluids dissolves, and allows the flukes to complete their life cycle. She says that a growth factor called ortho-phosphotyrosine (OPT), one of 25 recognized cancer-markers, stimulates normal cells that have been weakened by stress to go into unlimited division. Unless the body gets rid of this parasite-spawning chemical, excessive multiplication of cells takes over the tissues and cancer results.

This parasite doesn't have to stay in the intestines, but can be swept along in the bloodstream to lodge inside weakened tissues, such as benign breast lumps, smokers' lungs, and prostate glands saturated with mercury or other toxic metals. They grow fat in their new locations and stimulate cancer cell division.

In Southeast Asia intestinal flukes are transmitted when people bite into the unpeeled outer skin of plants that harbor the cyst form of this parasite. This includes the hulls of water chestnuts, bamboo shoots, and lotus plant roots.

Symptoms include diarrhea, nausea, ulceration, vomiting, abdominal pain and edema in the face and abdominal area. There can be intestinal obstructions, alternating diarrhea and constipation, vomiting, anorexia, edema of the face, abdominal wall, and legs, as well as retarded growth in children and occasionally anemia.

To confirm a diagnosis of intestinal flukes, there may be elevated white blood cells on a blood test, especially the eosinophils. On microscopic examination of the stool samples, there will be eggs present. Inflammation and ulceration of the intestinal wall are common findings.

To eliminate this infection in humans it is important to practice sanitary disposal of human feces. Dip aquatic plants in boiling water before eating. Conventional medicine recommends hexylresorcinol, tetrachlorethylene and praziquantel as the drugs of choice.

NANOPHYETUS SPP. (FISH-FLU FLUKE)

Nanophyetus salmincola or *Nanophyetus schikhobalowi* are the names of other North American and Russian flukes, but not much is known about these parasitic flatworms, often referred to as "fish flu" flukes. Infection from this fluke is transmitted by the cyst form in the flesh of freshwater fish. It can even survive the period spent at sea when it infects fresh water fish that also spend part of their lives in sea water. Although this cyst exists in many species of fish, it is usually transferred to humans in salmon and steelhead that are eaten raw, underprocessed, and smoked.

The illness in humans is characterized by an increase of bowel movements or diarrhea, abdominal discomfort, and nausea. Some people report weight loss and fatigue, and some are without symptoms. So far, there have been no major outbreaks from this parasite in North America. The only documented reports are of 20 cases coming from Oregon. A report in the popular press indicates that the frequency is significantly higher. Two cases occurred in New Orleans well outside the usual infection area. In Russia, the infection rate is reported to be greater than 90 percent and the size of the area where this parasite lives is growing.

An infection from this worm is usually accompanied by increased numbers of circulating eosinophils (a type of white blood cell). Detection of characteristic eggs in the feces is a positive diagnosis, but the eggs are difficult to distinguish from those of other parasites. Other tests may be available. The drug, mebendazole, was not that effective as a treatment since patients kept shedding eggs. But symptoms gradually decreased over the next two months or more. Treatment with two doses of bithionol or three doses of niclosamide resulted in the resolution of symptoms and the disappearance of eggs in the feces. These drugs are available in the United States from the Centers for Disease Control's Parasitic Drug Service. See "Resources" for the CDC's phone number.

PARAGONIMUS WESTERMANI (LUNG FLUKE)

Several species of lung flukes may infect humans, but this particular one is frequently involved. The adult lung fluke is a tiny, short and plump, reddish-brown flatworm that lives in the lungs of humans. Here they deposit their eggs where they are coughed up, and then either spit out or swallowed. If they are swallowed, they go through the intestines and pass out with the stool. When the eggs reach fresh water, they develop and enter a snail. Their life cycle continues as they pass from the snail to a crab.

When humans eat crayfish, freshwater crabs, or snails that are not cooked enough or eaten raw, the cyst form of these parasites enters the small intestines. The majority of the lung flukes continue their migration through the diaphragm and reach maturity in the lungs 5 to 6 weeks later. Some organisms stay in the intestines or wander to other areas of the body such as the liver, pancreas, kidney, skeletal muscle, under the skin, or into the central nervous system.

Lung flukes prefer to infect humans or wild carnivores, especially felines, but they will find rats, dogs, and pigs acceptable. Eating undercooked pork or leaving fresh crab juice on the kitchen surfaces can transmit this parasite to humans. Children living in areas where the lung fluke is endemic may be infected while playing with crabs. This parasite is most often found in Far Eastern nations such as Korea, China, Japan, Taiwan, the Philippines, and Indonesia, but it has recently been found in India, Africa, and Latin America.

The lung fluke can perforate and weaken the lungs and even cause oxygen starvation of the entire blood system. Once the lungs are weakened, it is easy to attract other illnesses, such as repeated flu and fungi infections. In a severe infection, a person can develop chronic pneumonia. Other symptoms include the occasionally mild cough and a peculiar bloodstained, brown, rusty sputum on awakening, along with an non-resolving lung abscess. This set of symptoms looks like tuberculosis. If the adult lung fluke enters the intestines, there can be symptoms of pain and bloody diarrhea, and on occasion produce abdominal masses. After lung flukes enter the brain, they can cause seizures similar to epilepsy or other central nervous system problems.

A diagnosis of lung flukes depends on these findings: signs similar to tuberculosis on x-ray; about half of the people with brain lesions will show calcification on x-ray of the skull; elevated eosinophils on blood test; detection of circulating antibodies; sputum or feces contains eggs. Eggs may not be seen in the sputum during the first 3 months of obvious infection. Repeated stool or sputum examinations will eventually produce the eggs in most infected people.

To prevent and control this organism there needs to be the proper disposal of feces and sputum; control snails; cook crabs and crayfish well before eating or handling them. Lightly salted, pickled, or wine immersion practices seldom kill this fluke. The disease responds well to the drugs bithionol or praziquantel.

SCHISTOSOMA SPP. (BLOOD FLUKE)

There are three primary species of blood flukes that cause disease. *Schistosomiasis mansoni* occurs in Africa, Eastern Mediterranean, the Caribbean, and South America; *Schistosomiasis japonicum* is found in Asia; and *Schistosomiasis haematobium* is found in Egypt. The disease caused by these blood flukes infect over 200 million people worldwide, in 71 countries. The widespread distribution and damage caused by this worm makes it the single most important worm infection in the world today. What keeps this blood fluke out of the continental United States is only the lack of a suitable snail host

When eggs are deposited in fresh water, the larvae hatch quickly and find a snail host particular to their species. After they invade the snail, this parasite is transformed over the next 1–2 months into thousands of forked-tail organisms. After leaving the snail, the infectious larvae swim about vigorously for a few days until they come into contact with human skin. Now they can attach themselves, discard their tails, and penetrate the skin.

After burrowing into the skin of humans, these flukes move through the bloodstream until the male attaches to the wall of a blood vessel by a sucker on his body. These tiny flatworms (1-2 centimeter long) typically stay in pairs of a male and a female. The male holds the longer and more slender female in a deep groove on his body for a life-long copulatory embrace. Each mating pair produces 300 to 3,000 eggs daily for the remainder of their 4–35 year life span. After mating, they use their suckers to move through the bloodstream eventually reaching their site of attack. Some attack the lining of the intestine or liver, others attack the bladder, urinary tract, or other pelvic organs. This parasite is increasing, especially in the rural tropics where there are irrigation farmers.

There is usually a self-limiting, but very itchy skin rash immediately after the parasite penetrates human skin. As the worms migrate to the liver, the rash disappears and the infected person experiences fever, headache, and abdominal pain for 1–2 weeks. One to two months after the first exposure, people with severe infections develop a fever and symptoms that looks very similar to serum sickness. Other symptoms could include a cough, arthritis-like symptoms, swollen lymph glands, and diarrhea.

The severity of the illness correlates with the amount of worms invading the body. The signs and symptoms vary with infecting species, but complications of chronic disease can be most serious.

There could be a thickening of the intestinal or bladder wall, blood in the urine, incontinence, dysentery, and hypertension. Adults could also have blood clots.

The blood fluke produces an enzyme that destroys the protein in blood. They consume certain amino acids, especially arginine, from the host's blood, causing a protein imbalance. Overall, a person infected with blood flukes feels toxic. Where this worm deposits its eggs, hemorrhage of the intestines, urinary bladder, or lung can occur, as well as considerable trauma to these tissues, such as the formation of abscesses. The body's immune defenses will be activated to destroy this parasite, but by doing so it also causes tissue proliferation and repair that can lead to cancer. This is the theory that Dr. Hulda Clark, Ph.D., N.D., discusses in her book, *The Cure For All Cancers.*

To be sure of a diagnosis, a laboratory looks for eggs in the urine and stool. Sometimes, a biopsy needs to be performed. All varieties can cause elevated eosinophils (a type of white blood cell) on blood tests. A sigmoidoscopic examination reveals an inflamed colon and signs of hemorrhages. Because dead eggs may persist in the tissues for a long time after the death of the adult worms, active infection is confirmed only if the eggs are alive. There may be available skin and blood tests to detect the presence of an active infection.

It is expensive and difficult to control this deadly disease. More modern construction of sanitation and water purification facilities would break this cycle of transmission. There needs to be health education to keep infected urine and feces out of the water supplies. Often antihistamines and corticosteroids may be helpful in stopping the more severe manifestations. The drug praziquantel is effective against all three species of schistosomes; metrifonate and oxamniquine may be useful for some species. Many of the drugs effective to kill this parasite are also very toxic to humans and the environment.

CHAPTER 7

Animal Care

When given a choice, it is always better to prevent parasites than wait until your pet is already infected. Many parasites are not that easy to get rid of. Unfortunately, most of this country's companion animals (dogs, cats, birds, and hamsters) already are common hosts to numerous and different parasites, and it is possible for you and your children to become infected. Do you sleep with your pet? Do your children pet animals and then put their hands in their mouth without washing them? Most people know that dogs and cats can transmit diseases by scratches and bites, but few people realize that close contact with pets, including handling animal fur, sleeping with your pet, and nuzzling, can cause serious illness.

The disease toxoplasmosis is usually acquired from cats and causes severe problems to the fetus in pregnant women. Infections from dog and cat roundworms can become severe and even life threatening, especially if a person also has a compromised immune system. The problems that come from the infestation of these parasites are usually unsuspected, even by the medical profession.

Your pet's parasites can exist on the outside and on the inside of the body. Many species of parasites are specific to only one type of animal, or they can exist on several different types of animals, regardless of their age. The greatest frequency occurs in puppies, kittens, and other young animals. This is probably because of their immature immune system. The type of parasite, and how dangerous it is, also depends on where you live.

Some tapeworms are visible to the naked eye, but they are hard to find. You could see their eggs if they consistently shed them in the feces. Certain intestinal parasites are only one-celled organisms, such as protozoans, and cannot be seen without the aid of a microscope. Most cases of pet-to-human transfer of parasites are prevented by simple measures, such as practicing good personal hygiene, eliminating intestinal parasites from the pets, and making potentially contaminated environments off limits to your children. Usually, pet owners have no idea that their friendly dog, adorable cat, or kissing bird can pass parasites to them. Therefore, pet owners do not take precautionary measures.

Talk to your veterinarian about treatment. They can provide important information about this problem by recommending well-timed deworming and other antiparasitic treatments. By counseling you on the potential for illness from parasites, your veterinarian can provide an important service. There are many things you can do to reduce the risk of you and your family contracting parasites from your pets:

- Check your pets routinely for worms and treat if needed. Tapeworm eggs look like white, rice-like particles. Pumpkin seed-like particles found on or near your dog are signs of dog tapeworm.
- Only give your pet cooked meat or dry food, not raw or undercooked meats. If your cats are outdoors eating birds and rodents, they will need to be dewormed on a regular basis.
- Clean and disinfect your pet's eating and drinking dish in hot soapy water regularly or sterilize it in the dishwasher.
- Do not let your pets get on the kitchen counter where you prepare food for eating. Keep your pets away from all areas designated for food preparation, and don't let them eat from your dishes.
- Keep your pet's sleeping areas clean.
- Don't allow your pets to defecate on lawns and playgrounds or in sandboxes where children play or other people would come in contact with the feces. Keep sandboxes covered. Collect and discard your animal's droppings. Burn the feces or put in the garbage for disposal. Do not flush down the toilet. Many parasites can survive in the sewage system.
- Empty the kitty litter box as often as possible; daily is best. You should wear gloves when handling soiled kitty litter. Concerned

pet owners should collect their pet's feces every day and burn them or place them in the garbage. Disinfect litter pans with boiling water and a mild bleach solution.

- If you have toddlers in the house, it is best to keep outdoor pets outside. An indoor pet is unlikely to pick up an infection since there is probably not a ready source of the parasite's eggs indoors.
- It is important to deworm all kittens and puppies, as well as grown pets on a regular basis. Some veterinarians suggest beginning at six weeks for kittens and two weeks for puppies, and routinely deworming adult dogs and cats every six months. Always consult your local veterinarian before deworming. Some dosages of medication depend on the weight of the pet and other requirements.
- Have your veterinarian check your pets for roundworm and tapeworm infestation. Parasites may be present if the animal shows signs of illness or is rubbing its anus against the carpet or floor. Also have your pets checked for other parasites.
- You need to deal with any flea problem, because they are carriers of tapeworms.
- Teach your children not to put their hands in their mouth after touching their pet or anything outside. If your pets play in the yard, this is a good place to pick up parasite eggs. Always have children wash their hands after playing outside, especially after playing with pets and soil.
- Wash hands on the top and bottom with soap and water after playing with a pet. Keep a nail brush by the sink and brush under the nails.
- Don't walk barefoot around animals. Exposed areas of the skin are a good way to acquire parasites.
- Stop kissing your pet whether it be a dog, cat, gerbil, or exotic bird. It is just as important not to let them kiss or lick you.
- Educate yourself about the risk and appropriate control measure concerning parasites

PROTOZOANS

One common intestinal parasite that occurs with some frequency is *Coccidia*, a one-celled protozoan. Infection occurs when a dog or puppy eats contaminated feces or food. Some adult dogs do not have any symptoms and the infection resolves on its own. Other dogs have diarrhea or bloody stools. Puppies are commonly at the highest risk for infection. In kennel environments, prevention is essential.

Usually a good steam cleaning of the kennels will eliminate the infestation. When the environment is difficult to control, add the medication to the food or water, especially for late stage pregnant dogs or young pups 3–6 weeks of age. Coccidia of dogs is usually not a threat to humans.

Cryptosporidium, a tiny protozoan, can be difficult to confirm on routine microscopic fecal exams. Special stains are required. The organism infects humans, cats and dogs. Puppies are primarily at risk and likely to show symptoms. The disease produces voluminous watery diarrhea that varies with the severity of the organism and the health of the host. Dogs who have compromised immune systems are at severe risk. The disease usually presents without symptoms or is self-limiting. Antibiotics may have some effect, but treatment is usually to combat fluid loss. Check with your veterinarian for current treatment.

Giardia is another intestinal protozoan that infects many animals including humans. The disease produced is variable depending on the animal and its age. Young animals are most often affected. Symptoms usually occur 1–2 weeks after infection and often the disease goes unnoticed or is self-limiting after a bout of diarrhea. It can produce severe diarrhea and fluid loss. Confirming that the parasite is giardia can be demanding and it may require several stool specimens. It does respond very well to treatment unless it is a resistant strain.

TAPEWORMS

The most common form of tapeworm is transmitted when a flea eats the egg of the tapeworm, and then the flea is eaten by a dog or cat. Humans occasionally get these tapeworms by ingesting a flea, too. Since humans pick fleas off rather than lick them off, we are spared getting tapeworms in this way. The eggs are not directly infective, but they do last a while in the environment, possibly as long as 15 months. It is a good idea to regularly vacuum and throw out the vacuum cleaner bag each time, at least for the next couple of times. Controlling the fleas in the house and on the pets will eliminate the spread of tapeworms. Young children are at a much higher risk because of their close contact with their pets.

Tapeworms in dogs are less common than in cats. The common tapeworms of dogs, cats, and other meat eaters, *Dipylidium caninum* and *Taenia pisiformi*, can be passed to humans. Eggs are shed into the environment from the animal in small segments that look like small pieces of rice. You can see these segments in fresh feces or attached to the area around the animal's anus. As the segments disintegrate, they release microscopic eggs into the environment for the cycle to begin again. Mature adult parasites can reach great lengths, but often the animal shows no symptoms of infestation, except the potential of further debilitation in an already compromised pet. Prevention of *Dipylidium* consists of good flea control. Prevention of *Taenia* is difficult if your dog is a good rodent and rabbit hunter and may require deworming several times a year.

ROUNDWORMS

The roundworms most often associated with pets are *Toxocara canis* and *Toxocara cati* (dog and cat roundworm). These common parasites can be transmitted to humans. They live and grow in an animal's intestines and reach lengths of up to 7 inches. The vast majority of infections occur in dogs when the parasite migrates from the pregnant female's uterus to the unborn pup. It has been speculated that 85 percent of puppies are infected with them. Therefore, it is important to begin deworming pups at 2 weeks of age and every 2 weeks until they are about 3 months old.

Cats do not seem to transfer roundworm infections to kittens in the uterus the way dogs do. Deworming begins in kittens at about 6 weeks of age, since it takes about that long for the infection to reach the stage where deworming medications are effective. Continue to deworm kittens every 2 weeks until they are about 4 months old. Once the initial infection is treated properly it is a good idea to occasionally check a stool sample for the presence of worms or to consider a course of deworming medications if the situation seems to warrant it, especially in outdoor cats and dogs.

Since many pups and kittens are not brought to a veterinarian before 6–8 weeks of age, treatment for parasites is usually delayed. By then the infection may be severe and even life-threatening. Because young animals acquire new parasite infections continuously from their mother's milk and from the environment, lab tests for these worms may be negative at the time of testing.

Effective worming medication is the best way to prevent the continuation of parasites in your pets and environment. All female dogs should be presumed carriers of roundworms even if they test negative. The larvae can remain "dormant" in tissues until the dog is pregnant. Adult male dog infections are estimated to be around 10-15 percent in this country.

When animals suffer from heavy roundworm infection, they appear potbellied, the coat is dull, and there may be vomiting and diarrhea. Lung and liver damage could occur. Roundworms can be serious in young animals producing abdominal pain, bloating, and occasionally fatal small bowel obstruction. There can be respiratory symptoms that mimic upper respiratory infections. Occasionally, a serious form of pneumonia results. Adult dogs rarely show digestive signs but this parasite can compromise their overall condition, especially if other diseases are active.

Roundworm migration of the larvae goes through the liver, diaphragm, lungs, and up the major airways. As the worm moves up the trachea, occasionally several worms will be coughed up by the young animal. Most of these organisms will continue their migration and be swallowed, moving down the esophagus, into the stomach and back into the small intestine where they reach adult breeding status and begin shedding eggs. Some of the migrating larvae will develop into a cyst in the tissues, remaining there without consequence during the dog's life. Most adult animals develop some immunity to reinfection.

When roundworms migrate in human tissue (larva migrans) the symptoms depend on the organs the parasite enters. The common parasite of dogs, *Toxocara canis,* has long been recognized as a cause of "larva migrans syndrome" in children. *Toxocara cati* from cats can also cause disease in humans, although for reasons partly related to the toilet behavior of cats, it does so less frequently. The larvae migrate through the human liver, lungs, and other organs and tissues where they produce damage and induce allergic responses. Infection may leave children with permanent visual or neurologic damage. *Toxocara canis* presents a serious threat when the larvae enter vital tissues, especially the eye. Children are at the greatest risk because they tend to put their fingers into their mouth without washing first. The high incidence, and the seriousness of this infection in children, makes it necessary to deworm family pets.

HOOKWORMS

Hookworms are common parasites of many animals, regardless of age. They are most common in warm humid climates, but exist all over North America. Just under 20 percent in all ages of dogs are infected, with symptoms ranging from no symptoms at all to severe ones. The worms are transmitted to animals when immature larvae penetrate the skin or by ingestion of contaminated feces. After the larvae penetrate the skin, they migrate into the bloodstream and are carried into many tissues. Most of them end up in the lungs, and like roundworms, are swallowed back into the intestinal tract. As mature hookworms, they attach to the lining of the intestinal tract and suck blood.

Hookworm larvae also migrate into the developing pup fetus and continue to mature when the pup is born. Puppy hookworm can be profound and require strong supportive care. Severe hookworm infection can cause marked anemia, intermittent bloody diarrhea, dull dry hair coat, and weight loss. Young and adult dogs that have compromised immune systems, or suffer with another disease, are at the highest risk.

As with roundworms, the migrating larvae require several dewormings given at 2–3 week intervals. Be sure you get your pet an annual fecal exam, but repeat more often if you live in a warm and humid climate. You could do a monthly worming in conjunction with preventing heartworm. It is also important to regularly remove and dispose of animal feces. Use a disinfectant such as bleach for cement dog runs. Treatment of lawns with a commercial product to kill the larvae of hookworms may also be necessary if repeated infections occur. To prevent the transmission of hookworms from pets to people it is important to practice good hygiene and sanitation, and provide well-timed preventive treatments, especially for puppies and kittens. Studies have implicated the presence of dogs, particularly puppies, as the principal risk factors for human disease from this parasite.

WHIPWORMS

Whipworms are commonly found in warm and humid climates, and are much less prevalent in the western dry areas of North America. It is difficult to diagnose this parasite and can take several fecal samples to find the egg in a microscopic exam. Symptoms usually include straining, mucus-filled diarrhea with occasional blood, and an urge to defecate frequently, but only small volumes of stool. Several treatments for whipworms are required. Severe cases of whipworms are not common, but have been known to require surgical intervention. Prevention includes careful removal of feces and bleaching dog runs regularly.

FLUKES

Existing only in the Northwest, *Nanophyetus salmincola* is a small intestinal fluke acquired by dogs when they consume raw salmon. The parasite is mostly harmless, but within the parasite lives a more serious threat. Many of the flukes are infected with *Neorickettsia helminthoeca,* a rickettsia that causes fever, anorexia, vomiting, diarrhea and death in up to 90 percent of the cases. Therapy involves supportive care including intravenous fluids and antibiotics. Prevention involves avoidance of raw freshwater fish.

CHAPTER 8

Laboratory Analysis for Parasites

More and more physicians are called upon to evaluate cases of persistent diarrhea and non-specific gastrointestinal symptoms in their patients. Intestinal parasites represent one possibility, but doctors usually do not consider this as the underlying cause. Even if the doctor does test for parasites, the results often come back negative, especially if only one stool sample is used. Then it is assumed that the patient does not have any parasites.

The diagnosis of most parasitic infections is dependent upon the laboratory. For intestinal parasites, the usual method has been the identification under a microscope of the egg, cyst, or adult parasite. This has always been an inadequate way to diagnose these organisms. Most laboratories fail to find the majority of intestinal parasites in stool specimens submitted to them for examination. Testing for intestinal parasites can be tricky, resulting in many false negatives. Testing for parasites in other parts of the body can be even more difficult. Some of the commercial labs simply don't have the facilities to do a very good job.

There have been cases when 12 or more stool samples had to be submitted before giardia could be confirmed by standard laboratory analysis. Many typical laboratories fail to diagnose parasitic infections because they rarely allow the time for careful analysis or multiple procedures. Most tests are performed on a single stool specimen, rather than on multiple stool samples gathered over several days. Diagnosis of some parasites by standard microscopic exam can be problematic because the evidence of parasites is often not in every stool sample, or there are so few organisms it is easy to miss them. Unfortunately, many parasites remain undetected.

In the cases of 125 people infected with *Entamoeba histolytica* or *Dientamoeba fragilis,* 13 percent of the stool samples had at least one of these parasites, if there was only one sample tested. If two samples were tested then the percentage of positive samples went up to 19 percent. Three samples jumped up to 65 percent, and more than three samples were needed for another increase of 6 percent. Thirteen people with *Entamoeba histolytica* required anywhere from 4 to 9 stool examinations before the parasite could be absolutely detected.

Tests for parasites should be done in a laboratory that specializes in parasitology to insure a better chance of detection. Even with the best laboratories, and with a patient suspected of having giardia, this organism shows up less than 50 percent of the time when one stool sample is used. When there is an increase from a single specimen to multiple specimens, detection increases to more than 95 percent. In addition to formed stools as a specimen source, many authorities agree that purged samples (induced by oral purgatives) provide valuable specimens. One newer detection method incorporates the use of a rectal swab technique that samples mucus instead of stool. There are apparently higher numbers of organisms in rectal mucus, making them easier to see.

Organisms that do not have a cyst stage are harder to detect on laboratory analysis, especially in stool samples. A recent public health study indicated that many samples infected with the ameba, *Dientamoeba fragilis,* usually go undetected. Improved detection occurs when the laboratory uses the rectal swab technique. The microscopic examination of the sample also improves when using a fluorescent stain. Because this parasite lives so low in the intestinal tract, in the cecum and colon, this test appears to be a very efficient method of collecting samples.

Immunofluorescent staining is proving a useful tool for detecting parasites. This technique uses antibodies against parasites tagged with fluorescent dyes. This makes the parasites highly visible under the microscope. Computer enhanced video microscopy also aids the laboratory technician in identification and provides the physician with an actual picture of any organisms found. You may have to ask the laboratory if they use these tests, since many places still do not have them.

Some specialty laboratories have turned to various immunoassay tests. These techniques are becoming more available for the detection of parasites, both intestinal and blood-borne, by checking for antibodies to the parasites. One test can pinpoint the presence of an antibody in most blood samples, while some detect antigens or use nucleic probes. Detection by immunoassay is not dependent on the presence of parasites in the stool, and testing on multiple stool specimens becomes unnecessary. Accuracy exceeds that of the traditional egg and parasite exam by 30–50 percent or more.

The diagnosis of parasites outside the intestinal tract is more difficult, since the parasite usually cannot be recovered from stool or tissue. Blood tests are of paramount importance in these cases. Typically, if the person does not have symptoms there is not any antibody production. In most people with symptoms, the immune system comes into play, resulting in a diagnostic titer. Unfortunately, these titers may persist for months to years after an acute infection, making the interpretation of a positive test difficult in areas where the parasite is endemic.

At present, the indirect hemagglutination test and the ELISA assay appear to be the most sensitive. Several rapid tests, including latex agglutination and counter-immuno-electro-phoresis are available to smaller laboratories. There may be other tests available as well. It makes sense that the more sophisticated the detection procedures, the higher the percentage of detection.

In the country of Brazil, there were tests done to see what the prevalence of intestinal parasites was in food handlers. They looked at 20 different public elementary schools in various areas of a city. Stool samples were collected from 104 cooks and their helpers, who were working in some area of food preparation. They were all females between the ages of 24 and 69 years. Intestinal parasites were found in 47 percent of the food handlers. Among the infected, 65 percent carried a single parasite and 35 percent carried two parasites. Would we see these kinds of results in this country? Since this kind of testing is not commonly done here, it is hard to know just how prevalent parasites really are in the people who handle our food. The following intestinal parasites were most often found:

- *Giardia lamblia* 21.1 percent
- *Entamoeba coli* 21.1 percent
- *Necator americanus* 9.6 percent

- *Ascaris lumbricoides* 5.8 percent
- *Entamoeba histolytica* 2.9 percent
- *Hymenolepis nana* 1.9 percent
- *Strongyloides stercoralis* 1.0 percent

Another group studied pinworm infection for one year in 469 children attending three day-care centers in this country. Each child was examined at six-month intervals using up to three peri-anal swabs with adhesive tape. At the beginning of the study they found 28 percent of the children had parasites. The reinfection rate was just as high.

In 1990, a laboratory that specializes in parasites analyzed 67 people from around the country. Fifty-one of them turned out to be infested with at least one parasite that causes chronic gastrointestinal symptoms. The findings were confirmed by the Parasitic Diseases Division of the United States Center for Disease Control and Prevention. These people had all been seeking medical treatment for their chronic digestive complaints of diarrhea with abdominal pain.

Even though most public health laboratories are not that accurate with parasite tests, a survey of public health laboratories still found almost 16 percent of the examined specimens contained at least one parasite. Other nonspecialty parasitic labs commonly found 20 percent of the specimens examined positive for parasites. These figures are probably low because many people are never tested for parasites in the first place. In a 1994 study, the Institute of Parasitic Diseases tested 188 patients for intestinal parasites. The following parasites occurred in these percentages:

- 53 percent had *Blastocystis hominis*
- 26 percent had some form of ameba
- 14 percent had *Giardia lamblia*
- 8 percent had *Cryptosporidium parvum*
- 19 percent had some form of roundworm
- 12 percent had some form of tapeworm

Another study examined 321 stool samples from children. Intestinal parasites were present in 49 percent. Multiple parasitic species were present in 20 percent of the children with a positive stool specimen. There were not any significant differences between the positive or negative stools with regard to age, sex, ethnic group, monthly income, or number of people in a household. The most significant correlation was that most of the people diagnosed with parasites had recently traveled.

A comprehensive review was done of all stool examinations performed at a children's hospital in Canada during a 3-year period. A total of over 1,500 children were surveyed. Eighty-five percent of the children were infected with a single parasite. A much smaller number had two or more parasites. The following parasites were found:

* *Giardia lamblia* 31 percent
* *Dientamoeba fragilis* 23 percent
* *Entamoeba coli* 16 percent
* *Blastocystis hominis* 13 percent
* *Cryptosporidium parvum* 8 percent
* *Endolimax nana* 4 percent
* *Enterobius vermicularis* 2 percent
* *Hymenolepis nana* 2 percent
* *Iodamoeba buetschlii* 1 percent

After completing an apparently effective treatment program, it is important to be retested. It is advisable to continue the treatment regimen until at least two parasite tests, performed one month apart, are negative. When being retested, it is always a good idea to inquire if any new methods of detection are being used. The following laboratories specialize in the detection of parasites:

The Great Smokies Diagnostic Laboratory
18A Regent Park Boulevard
Asheville, North Carolina 28806
(800) 522-4762
This company employs the highest quality and broadest range of detection methods and equipment available for comprehensive parasitology testing. These is also a detoxification profile available that assesses the body's capacity to carry out detoxification showing the body's capacity and potential for damage. They provide collection kits, articles, abstracts and other publications regarding their testing methodology, clinical applications and patient aids. Great Smokies Diagnostic Laboratory is committed to increasing the scientific and public knowledge of parasites for healthcare providers and the public.

The Center for the Improvement of Human Functioning
International, Inc.
3100 North Hillside Avenue
Wichita, Kansas 672191
(800) 447-7276
This Bio-Center Laboratory provides diagnostic services for physicians throughout the United States.

Medical Diagnostic Laboratory
3250 Westchester Avenue
Bronx, New York 10461
(212) 828-1500
Offers comprehensive parasitological testing.

Institute of Parasitic Diseases (IPD)
Diagnostic and Educational Laboratory
3530 E. Indian School Road, Suite 3
Phoenix, Arizona 85018
(602) 955-4211 Fax (602) 955-4102
This is a diagnostic and educational laboratory for the detection of
parasites. The director is Dr. Omar M. Amin, Ph.D. He was a pro-
fessor of parasitology and epidemiology at the University of
Wisconsin and is currently a professor of parasitology at Arizona
State University. Dr. Amin has over 100 major articles/book chapters
published in the U.S. and foreign professional journals on human
and animal parasites from North America, Peru, North Africa, the
Persian Gulf, Kenya, Czechoslovakia, Russia, China, Taiwan and
India.

CHAPTER 9

Water Filters

Water supply sources, including both ground and surface water, are being contaminated and endangered by harmful organisms. Ground water includes underground aquifers, wells or springs. They provide water to about one-half the population. Surface waters, such as ponds, rivers, and lakes, serve as the water source for the rest of the population. The dumping of animal and human waste onto the soil affects both water sources.

Millions of people may be needlessly exposed to unhealthy drinking water. In one of the most comprehensive drinking water studies ever, the Natural Resources Defense Council analyzed Environmental Protection Agency (EPA) records and found in 1991-1992 that 43 percent of all water suppliers violated federal health standards. Less than 40 percent of the water treatment plants in the United States effectively removes organisms such as cryptosporidium.

The water supply infrastructure does not seem capable of providing safe water consistently in many areas of this country. Usually, the larger municipal water-treatment systems that supply more than 100,000 customers have the resources to keep up with EPA standards. Small water systems serving less than 3,500 people usually have neither the technology nor the resources to keep pace. In a recent study, 92 percent of the small water systems were in violation of EPA standards.

The chlorination and filtering of a municipal water-treatment plant can work properly and you can still get ill. It was reported in the *American Journal of Public Health*, 1991, that over 600 households in a Montreal suburb experienced gastrointestinal symptoms including nausea, vomiting, diarrhea, cramps, muscle pains, colds, sore throats, and fever. The water had met all current water quality criteria by the state and federal government, yet people still got sick. It was thought that the contaminate was a parasite.

If the EPA doesn't test for a substance or an organism, or if they don't consider it harmful, it is possible to find it in the water. What is considered safe drinking water today may not be considered safe tomorrow if the EPA enacts new standards. Remember, "safe" is EPA standards, and may not meet your personal standards for healthy drinking water.

From the years 1971 to 1985, the Center for Disease Control says that an average of 7,400 cases of illness in the United States can be linked to drinking water. These figures are probably very low, since many illnesses are never blamed on the water source. From 1971 to 1990, according to the EPA, over 140,000 people in the United States became ill as a result of 570 documented cases of contaminated water. For each illness reported, it is thought that at least 25 probably go unreported.

Chlorine does not rid the water supply of many harmful organisms. Microorganisms such as protozoa, fungi, viruses, and coliform bacteria have been found alive and flourishing in chlorinated tap water. These organisms are potentially dangerous to anyone who consumes them. They are especially dangerous to people with weakened immune systems such as those receiving chemotherapy, radiation therapy, and those who have AIDS. Chlorine also does not kill other pathogens, including the one that causes the pneumonia known as Legionnaires' disease. Almost all recent outbreaks of Legionnaires' disease were traced to water-distribution systems.

Tap water, mountain streams, and well water, are prime sources of contamination by *Giardia lamblia*. Outbreaks can hospitalize hundreds of people because of severe gastrointestinal symptoms. The protozoan, *Cryptosporidium muris,* is transmitted through contaminated ground water, farm animals, and the fecal-oral route. It also causes gastrointestinal symptoms especially diarrhea. While most water systems may effectively filter out giardia cysts, the cryptosporidium cysts are so tiny, only 0.02 millimeters in diameter, that they are not filtered out. This makes them especially difficult to eliminate.

Not only do most filtering systems not working adequately, but the added chlorine does not kill cryptosporidium and may not kill giardia. The only reliable way to insure that these cysts do not end up in your drinking water is to use adequate filtration. Water systems that were built before the late 1970s did not know that cryptosporidium cysts were a problem to filter out. In April of 1993, over 370,000 residents of Milwaukee found out what this means. They became ill, and at least 40 were killed from the contamination by cryptosporidium. It entered the water supply through fecal material from an upstream dairy farm, but the city's treatment system did not filter out this pathogen. It is hard to detect, and harmful strains are not easily distinguishable from the harmless.

Some people believe that they are safe because their water comes from a well or from the lake where they live. You couldn't be more wrong. The surrounding land at your well site may have the animal waste seeping into your water supply. Contaminated ground water from any source can affect rural area wells. If you want to be sure that you will have water that is safe to drink, then add a good filtration system.

The best filtering systems will remove virtually any health hazard from your drinking water. But there are currently many water filtration systems being sold that are totally inadequate, removing little of the unhealthy substances. Buying the best system that you can is a small price to pay when considering the alternative. Filtering your water is far more advantageous than the price you pay for bottled water. How do you know what has been filtered out or killed in the bottled water? There is not any labeling to tell how the water was processed. To guarantee clean, contaminant-free water, you will have to take matters into your own hands, and you easily can. Systems combining several features are often necessary. Common equipment choices include:

Carbon Filters

Most of the home water-treatment devices found on today's market are simple carbon filters. They come in sizes that can be mounted at the faucet or under the counter. In general, carbon filters work best at removing odors, chlorine, bad taste, organic chemicals, and pesticides. They may be more effective when used in conjunction with reverse osmosis or distillation.

The simplest and least expensive way to filter your water is to use activated charcoal. It will remove organic chemicals, pesticides, some heavy metals, and improve the taste of the water. These filters are less effective against microorganism contamination and heavy metals. They will not remove most minerals. Activated charcoal filters are inexpensive and do not require electricity to filter the water. All you have to do is just turn on the tap. Charcoal filters must contain a fine pore filter that exceeds no more than three microns in size. They also must be replaced regularly to maintain good water quality. If you do not change the filters frequently, bacteria will grow on the carbon. Cheap faucet-mounted carbon filters may become contaminated within days of use. Using higher volume models that fit under the counter cost more.

Some charcoal units are impregnated with silver to inhibit bacteria growth. The addition of silver does not improve the ability of the unit to physically remove bacteria or other contaminants, especially chemicals. Studies on the effectiveness of bacteriostatic filters have not shown promising results regarding their ability to control bacterial growth.

Bone carbon or hydroxyapatite charcoal is better at absorbing heavy metals and toxic minerals from the water. In order for the carbon filter to remain effective and not further contaminate the water, clean the filters of the algae, mildew, and other life forms that collect on it. Back-washing removes this residue very effectively

CARBON BLOCK FILTER

The carbon block filter is better than just using a simple carbon filter. It is more densely packed with a finer carbon that traps even smaller particles and some toxic metals. It removes most bacteria, organic chemicals, and some toxic metals, but allows some minerals to pass through the carbon block. Different stages of carbon remove different size particles.

The nationally recognized standards established for the drinking water treatment industry confirm that the most effective systems for the removal of contaminants are those that use solid carbon block filtering technology. This type of filter does a better job, but is more expensive than simple carbon. It still must be changed often, can grow bacteria, and does not remove all the toxic metals. If you do not replace the filter often enough, it can dump the accumulated toxic matter back into your filtered water.

Distillation Method

If your purpose is the removal of lead and other heavy metals, distillers offer the best choice. This method involves boiling water and then recondensing it. It produces a very pure, mineral-free, bacteria-free water. A problem with this method is that organic chemicals boil at a lower temperature than water. When the water recondenses, the organic chemicals can return to the purified water. Solve this problem with a fractional distilling system or use a carbon filter. Some systems double boil to remove the organic chemicals. At least no toxic substances exist in distilled water.

One of the main disadvantages of the distillation method is that it leaves a flat taste that many people don't like, unless a little air is mixed with the water. It also uses electricity and so has a higher cost than some other systems. You must clean them after every use, and it takes an hour or so to produce a gallon of water.

Not everyone wants to remove all the minerals from their drinking water, because they are beneficial when in reasonable balance. If you choose to drink distilled water to the exclusion of all other liquids, then you should supplement your diet or water with extra minerals to make up for the poor supply. Otherwise, this may produce serious health hazards. For short-term, detoxification purposes, distilled water is usually not a problem.

Reverse Osmosis Method

This cleans out lead, nitrates, pesticides, and many organic compounds by forcing water through microscopically fine screens. They are effective, but use up to six gallons of water to produce one drinkable gallon. Reverse osmosis involves forcing water through a semipermeable plastic membrane that allows only the water to pass through. The purified water is then passed through a carbon filter to eliminate any gases and other volatile chemicals, as well as removing minerals and organic compounds.

Combined with a charcoal filter, the reverse osmosis method provides one of the best filtering systems available today. Reverse osmosis is now the industry standard for water purification. They are available in under-the-sink and counter-top units. They produce almost distilled-quality water without using extra electricity. The filters operate as long as there is adequate water pressure.

The main disadvantages of reverse osmosis systems are having to change the membrane and carbon filters regularly. Since the membrane is back-washed to prevent clogging, some water is wasted. It uses three to six gallons of water for every gallon of drinking water produced and requires an hour or more to produce a gallon of water. These systems usually cost more than carbon filters and other simple devices. Some reverse osmosis devices may be ineffective at removing high levels of hard minerals such as calcium and magnesium.

Of all the water-purification systems available, reverse osmosis furnishes the purest and best-tasting liquid product, without the flat taste of distilled water. This is because they release extra oxygen molecules during the purification process. If you are drinking reverse osmosis filtered water you will need to supplement your diet with extra minerals, since it also has a poor supply. One brand, Multi-Pure, does not remove the natural minerals and does not waste water.

Bottled and Spring Water

You can buy a variety of sources from your local supermarkets. The water quality varies depending on the source. They are often high in minerals. This is fine as long as they don't include toxic metals. You can't tell from the label what type of filtration has been used so you don't really know how pure the water is. Hopefully, it does not contain any pesticides, nitrates, or high levels of bacteria. Some food markets have facilities so that you can buy purified or filtered drinking water. It is usually inexpensive, but how do you know when the filters were last changed, or what kinds of filter are being used? Some bottled drinking water has fluoride added in.

The latest information suggests that some bottled water may have higher-than-acceptable levels of bacteria. The economics of filtering your own water is far more advantageous than buying bottled water, and you know it is safe.

You may choose from many drinking water systems. With more than 500 companies selling treatment products, it is hard to compare one product to another. The EPA does not establish standards or testing protocol for devices used to treat drinking water. They refer consumers seeking information to NSF International. This is an organization devoted to developing and administering programs related to public health. These are international standards for consumer products and services, including drinking water treatment units. They provide assurance to the consumer that filtering devices certified by them will perform according to the claims made by the manufacturer or distributor. NSF has two standards that apply to devices used to filter drinking water:

1) Aesthetic Effects (NSF Standard No. 42)

These are claims for taste, odor, color, and other aesthetic effects, including the reduction of chlorine and particulate matter. Different classes define the level of chlorine and particulate reduction. The classes are:

• Taste, Odor and Chlorine Reduction
Class I reduces chlorine by 75 percent to 100 percent
Class II reduces chlorine by 50 percent to 74 percent
Class III reduces chlorine by 25 percent to 49 percent

• Particulate Reduction
Class I—0.5 to 1 micrometers (sub micron)
Class II—1 to 5 micrometers (extra fine)
Class III—5 to 15 micrometers (medium fine)
Class IV—15 to 30 micrometers (fine)
Class V—30 to 50 micrometers (medium coarse)
Class VI—50 micrometers and larger (coarse)

2) Health Effects (NSF Standard No. 53)

These are claims for the reduction of specific contaminants from drinking water (public or private). These contaminants are considered potential health hazards. Such hazardous contaminants may be microbiological, chemical, or particulate in nature, including filterable cysts. A unit may be effective in controlling one or more of these contaminants, but it is not a requirement that it control all of them. Included under this standard are:

• *Chemicals and Heavy Metals:* This includes chemical and heavy-metal contaminants such as lead, trihalomethanes, lindane, 2,4-D, asbestos, trichloroethylene, and others.
• *Volatile Organic Chemicals:* This includes 20 volatile organic contaminants.

- *Turbidity:* A condition caused by the presence of suspended particulate matter.
- *Cysts:* Tests determine the effectiveness of the unit in removing microscopic organisms such as *Giardia lamblia*.

When choosing a drinking-water system, you can use the NSF standards and listings to compare one device to another. In addition, the NSF standards also provide the basis for comparing the service life of the units and/or their replacement filters, as well as the flow rate of the device. The following important questions can help to evaluate any drinking water system:

1. Ask for the NSF listing for the specific product(s) you are evaluating. Is the product listed under NSF Standard No. 53 or under Standard No. 42?
2. Ask for the product performance data sheet. Many states require that performance data sheets be provided to all prospective customers of drinking water treatment devices.
3. Ask about the service cycle (stated in gallons of water treated) of the device. How often will you need to change the filter and what will replacement filters cost?
4. Ask about the range of contaminants that the unit can reduce under Standard No. 53. Be sure that the contaminants concerning you can be removed by the device you are considering. Most units certified under Standard No. 53 are listed for turbidity and cyst reduction only. Fewer units also reduce chemicals, lead, VOCs, and trihalomethanes.
5. Ask about the product's flow rate.
6. Ask if the manufacturer or distributor provides a customer satisfaction guarantee or warranty.

There are other things that you can do to protect yourself from parasites in the drinking water:

- Have your tap water tested. The EPA has a safe drinking water hotline that can give you more information on who to contact. Call (800) 426-4791.
- It is best to get in the habit of only drinking filtered water.
- Buy a unit that can filter the smallest possible organism so even the cysts of cryptosporidium can be filtered out. A fine pore filter of

not more than three microns is desirable. If you use a charcoal filter, it must contain a fine pore filter.

- Change the filter frequently to assure that the water will not be contaminated.
- Be sure that the water filtration unit that you buy is designed to block the microorganisms discussed in this book. Some companies have a microfiltration system specifically designed to block such microorganisms. New and improved methods of water purification are always coming out. Recently, I saw a unit that included ultra violet radiation and ozone as part of its package to kill organisms that slipped through the filtering system.
- Boil the water if you do not have any way of filtering out possible pathogens.
- If you spend time outdoors camping, hiking, swimming, etc., you should never drink our of the rivers and streams even if they look fresh and enticing. All outdoor water must be filtered, boiled, or treated in some way to address the possible contamination of parasites.

Be sure of the water you drink. Prevention beats a cure any day. If you are away from home and have doubts about the local water supply, bring or buy bottled water or bring the water to a boil for at least a minute. You can pick up water filters that filter out microorganisms at your local outdoor and camping stores. You can avoid water-borne diseases by paying careful attention to what you drink.

Consumers are often deceived by manufacturer's claims and the information, or lack of it, given by sales people. This makes it more important than ever to refer to industry standards and state regulation. You need to know if the effectiveness of the drinking-water systems has been certified or registered in reducing the substances and/or contaminants that you are paying for. To receive more information on drinking water and equipment, you can contact the following:

National Sanitation Foundation
3475 Plymouth Road
P.O. Box 1468
Ann Arbor, MI 48105

Water Quality Association
4151 Naperville Road
Lisle, IL 60160
(708) 505-0160

EPA Drinking Water Hotline
(800) 426-4791
call (202) 382-5533 in Alaska
and the District of Columbia

The following mail-order laboratories offer a variety of home water-testing options and prices:

National Testing Laboratories
6151 Wilson Mills Road
Cleveland, OH 44143
(800) 458-3330

Suburban Water Testing Labs
4600 Kutxtown Road
Temple, PA 19560
(800) 433-6595

Water Test
33 South Commercial St.
Manchester, NH 03101
(800) 426-8378

CHAPTER 10

Internal Body Clean-up

The body is designed to convert and neutralize the body's toxins into safe by-products ready for elimination. Many things interfere with this process increasing the detoxification burden. They include repeated exposure to chemicals and environmental pollution, lack of exercise, poor air quality, and emotional stress. The body is constantly being given additives and preservatives, as well as toxic substances that occur naturally when food is not completely digested and allowed to putrefy or ferment in the intestines. A person's lifestyle also plays a significant role. When you are infected with parasites, they also produce toxic waste material that adds to the overall load of toxins placed on the body.

The intestinal lining is your primary barrier to toxic compounds getting into the bloodstream. It is important to keep your intestines healthy or it can lead to an overload of these compounds entering the circulation and the liver's detoxifying system for processing and elimination. If the liver does not have the capacity to process these toxins, then they remain harmful to the body and depress the immune system. Now the detoxification system becomes even less efficient in ridding itself of these toxins and certainly places the body at a greater risk for damage.

WHY CLEANSE FIRST?

The main reason that it is so important to do a cleansing prior to starting a specific detoxification program is to minimize the adverse effects. If any symptoms do occur, they are usually mild, transient and self-limiting. A change in bowel function, flu-like reactions, headaches, and a lack of energy can be associated with detoxification. If the body has not been prepared to detoxify first, the resulting symptoms can be quite severe.

HOW OFTEN SHOULD I DETOXIFY?

After the initial process of cleansing, detoxification, and rebuilding, it is suggested that a yearly follow-up may be necessary. Have the sources of your toxins been eliminated? Have lifestyle changes been made? If you continue to be exposed to toxins, then you will need to repeat this treatment more frequently.

SUPPRESSING THE SYMPTOMS OF DETOXIFICATION

This process of detoxification is often mistaken for symptoms of disease. It is important to recognize the body's attempt to return to normal function by eliminating toxins. Instead, most people take something to stop the symptoms. This could be doing great harm by suppressing these vital eliminative functions. The body needs to eliminate toxins from the body or they will be reincorporated into new tissues and the toxic burden increases even more. Once the immune system recognizes these toxins as foreign then it may start a process of self-attack creating conditions such as "autoimmune" diseases or other illnesses.

Improve the Detoxification Process

The first step is to eliminate the sources of toxic exposure from the environment. Then you can assist the body's ability to eliminate both the parasite and the body's store of toxins with a program of cleansing, detoxification, and rebuilding.

I. CLEANSING PHASE

A. Preparing For Detoxification

It is important to have all the body's organs of elimination working properly so that they will be able to remove the toxins. Under ideal conditions this is what the body is designed to do: cleansing and detoxifying. To maintain a healthy environment for cell growth and body maintenance the body must eliminate these toxins. The five organs responsible for eliminating the body's waste products and toxins are: the skin, lungs, kidneys, intestines, and liver. A health program only works if your organs of elimination and excretion are fully functioning.

- The skin eliminates water, salts, and waste products. Keep it clean of dry dead skin cells so it will function properly. Use a loofah sponge when bathing because soap tends to block the pores. Dry brush the skin with a vegetable bristle brush, but always brush toward the heart.
- The lungs eliminate carbon dioxide and water. They function better with exercise. Develop a habit of doing 2 or 3 deep breaths before each meal, but avoid doing this in a smoky environment. A brisk daily walk is very beneficial.
- The primary organ of excretion are the kidneys. They eliminate salts, urea, uric acid, creatinine, metabolized hormones, and water. You have to drink adequate pure water each and every day. You could use distilled water that is free of all chemicals and minerals, but drink at least 6–8 glasses each day.
- The intestines eliminate roughage, water, salts, and dead cells. If the small intestines are building up excessive amounts of mucus from foods, absorption will be reduced, slowing down all nutrient utilization. The cleaner the small intestines, the faster any course of action will show results. Your diet should avoid foods such as salt, sugar, and milk products. To further reduce mucus make sure that at least 50 percent of your diet is from alkaline-forming foods. For more information on mucus-forming foods see my book *Allergies and Holistic Treatments*.
- Many toxins must be transformed by the liver from fat soluble to water soluble compounds before they can be eliminated by the kidneys. When the bowels become overloaded with toxins, the excess goes to the liver for detoxification. The liver is the primary storage organ for some toxins. If the liver becomes overburdened, the toxins spill over into the bloodstream.

The liver is equipped to handle most normal levels of toxin production. When an additional load occurs as a result of parasitic infestation, along with poor intestinal health, food allergies, and bacterial and yeast overgrowth, then the detoxification pathways can get overwhelm. Now the kidneys, lungs, and skin have to take up the job of cleansing. This added overload to the body can cause a host of symptoms creating various health situations.

B. Cleansing

The next step in getting rid of parasites is to cleanse the gastrointestinal tract. Some parasites live between the encrusted fecal material and the lining of the intestines where they are hard to reach. Until this built up encrusted material is eliminated, the parasites can hide from even effective medication. It is important to avoid foods that interfere with this process such as sugar, caffeine, chocolate, and fried foods. The toxins secreted by parasites in the body have to be eliminated as well. If your drink alcohol, smoke cigarettes, and eat junk food, you will over load the body's ability to detoxify.

Cleansing the intestines with herbal combinations can easily, safely and effectively rid your body of toxic waste. While doing any cleanse, some people experience nausea because toxins are being released too quickly and not being eliminated from the body adequately. Sometimes it is necessary to start slower or switch to a less powerful cleansing product.

This is where products containing substances such as psyllium husks, flaxseed, bentonite clay, oat products, guar gum, pectin, and papaya extract are effective. These substances help to dissolve and remove waste material from the intestines. It is important to establish regular bowel movements. Constipation invites parasites and makes it hard to release the toxins that have built up in the body. You should have at least two bowel movements a day before trying to kill off the parasites.

If there is poor peristaltic action in the large intestines, toxins will be reabsorbed. The longer the feces remain in the bowel, the more moisture is removed, resulting in hard stools, constipation, and hemorrhoids. A diet high in fiber will improve the movement of waste material, but you should increase fiber in the diet slowly, as well as increase the intake of water. Avoid over using fiber products since they bind minerals and prevent the absorption of key nutrients. Fiber induces mucus secretion in the bowels and reduces the attachment of parasites such as tapeworms. Intestinal cleansing and detoxifying products used in conjunction with colonics will remove encrustation rapidly, but without colonics, gradually. Use the minimal amount of supplements during the cleansing phase, but continue to support the organs of elimination.

C. Detoxification

This is when you take something to kill or stun the parasites and eliminate the toxins that they produce. Only start this phase after the previous steps have been accomplished. It may take several days or weeks before you are ready to begin the detoxification process. Now the body can release accumulated toxins from storage sites and subsequently send them to the kidney, liver, and other organs to be eliminated.

The die-off effects different people in different ways. People who have serious symptoms or who harbor a large viral or bacterial burden in their bodies may experience extreme fatigue, headaches, muscle/joint pain or flu-like symptoms that can begin almost immediately after treatment is started. These are really a positive response that the treatment is working, but you can still feel really rotten. This is because the body is now full of the dead organisms resulting in a variety of toxic symptoms.

If your body's ability to detoxify is impaired there are serious consequences. Free radical production can damage the body resulting in disorders such as allergies, fibromyalgia, chronic fatigue, and inflammatory joint disease. Lacking the critical nutrients needed for detoxification can contribute to chronic fatigue, environmental sensitivities or other chronic illnesses. This leaves fewer nutrients available for the body to rebuild its tissues.

It is very important during this process not to be on a reduced calorie program such as when trying to lose weight. Nutrient-dense unprocessed foods are absolute necessity to provide quantity protein, vitamins and minerals. Eat high-quality protein sources such as fish, eggs, beans or other legumes. Vegetarians need to concentrate on getting complete sources of protein. Keep up adequate pure water intake of at least 4–5 eight ounce glasses each day to promote elimination.

There are many products on the market for detoxification. I strongly recommend that you seek professional help from someone trained in this field. I have covered elsewhere in this book many of the herbs, supplements, and other products used to eliminate parasites from the body. As I have stated before, many of these products can be toxic and should be monitored by someone trained in their use.

D. Support

Eating healthy is recommended during both the cleansing and detoxification process. The body needs foods that are easy to digest and assimilate during both the cleansing and detoxification process, but it also needs foods that heal and do not harm the body.

It is most important to avoid junk foods of all kinds, including soft drinks, juices, as well as pork. Red meats, animal fats, sugar, and other simple and refined carbohydrates, salt, alcohol and caffeine should be avoided as much as possible. Avoid any foods that produce allergic reactions or other digestive problems.

You could include well-cooked fish, chicken, turkey and vegetable protein found in the different kinds of beans, and include vegetable-rich vitamin A foods. These are cooked sweet potatoes, carrots, and most green leafy vegetables. Eat with an emphasis on natural, organic, unrefined, and unprocessed foods prepared fresh from their natural state with a minimum of food additives and added chemicals. Fresh vegetables and fruits, whole grains, and unrefined starches need to be the majority of the diet. A balanced supply of nutrients should include about 60 percent of calories from complex carbohydrates, 20 percent from protein, and 20 percent from fat. Remember, raw foods are a source of parasites and need to be put in a food wash before eating. Otherwise, it is best to cook all foods before eating them during this time of cleansing and detoxification.

II. REBUILDING PHASE

The rebuilding phase begins after you have completed the cleansing and detoxification phases. Rebuild your system with a combination of live foods, vitamins and minerals, herbs, antioxidants, and digestive enzymes. This includes herbals, nutritional supplements, and other appropriate dietary supplements to support the body. This should include vitamin C. Many nutrients are in short supply in today's highly refined and nutrient-depleted diets. Adequate amounts of protein reduce a number of toxins.

It is important as part of the rebuilding phase to recolonize the intestinal tract with beneficial bowel flora. These include *Lactobacillus acidophilus,* and *Lactobacillus bifidus.* These friendly bowel organisms help to fight off foreign invaders and keep the proper pH in the intestinal tract, as well as producing important nutrients and certain enzymes. They also produce antibiotics and other antimicrobial substances that suppress the growth of pathogenic organism and reduce putrefaction and toxins. It is important to use a quality product that has been kept under refrigeration or you might find that there will not be any colonies of these beneficial bacteria produced.

Take on an empty stomach at least 30 minutes before eating and only with water.

How Much Should I Exercise?

Stretching exercises in combination with deep breathing is extremely effective as a method of stress reduction. Aerobic exercise at your target heart rate for 20 minutes every other day further reduces stress as well as your risk for heart disease and other chronic illnesses. Muscle building and strengthen training, especially of the lower body, is beneficial when combined with aerobic and stretching exercises. Activities such as walking, biking, and swimming are excellent. Active people have minimal problems with cleansing and detoxification.

What Are Colonics?

Colonics, or colon irrigation, is one of the important treatments available for a multitude of health problems. The usual colonic treatment lasts about 45 minutes. A small speculum is inserted into the person's rectum. The speculum is then attached to a plastic hose that connects to the colonic machine. The colonic therapist adjusts the volume and temperature of the water coming out of the machine that runs through a plastic hose into the person's rectum and through the entire colon. The person is temporarily filled with a certain volume of water to individual tolerance. This will induce peristaltic contractions in the colon. Now the person will begin to expel fecal matter through the colonic hose that leads back to the colonic machine and through a clear plastic viewing tube. Some of the things seen are mucus, parasites, and very old fecal material.

This old fecal material may have been lying in the person's colon for years. It looks like vulcanized rubber and has that kind of consistency. It is important to remember that it took years for the colon to become clogged up with its own waste products. The fecal encrustation interferes with healthy intestinal flora, peristaltic action for moving feces out of the body, and the absorption of nutrients coming into the colon from the small intestine. It should be noted that most people need a series of colonic irrigations, not just one. It usually takes a few treatments before the colon starts dislodging old encrusted fecal matter. When the bowel is toxic it can harbor an amazing variety of very harmful bacteria and parasites.

When you choose a colon therapist, be certain that they have received proper training and that the facility is clean and well maintained. Since fecal matter can transmit disease, it is most important that the equipment and the facility be thoroughly sterilized. They should be using disposable tubing and speculums so that contaminated equipment is never used from one person to the next. For sources of referral to a colon therapist ask your chiropractor, naturopathic physician, health food store, or other alternative clinics, or look in your local phone directory. Check "Resources" for agencies that have referrals to colonic therapists in your area.

CHAPTER 11

Medicinal Herbs

The majority of the world's population continues to use indige-
nous traditional medicines derived mainly from plants for the
treatment of disease. Plants have been used successfully for hundreds of years to kill and expel parasites. The basic protocol, besides
careful attention to hygiene and to provide an inhospitable diet to
the parasite, is to give botanical medicines to stun or poison. It is
also important to give a purgative or laxative, to expel the worm(s)
or other parasites from the intestinal tract. Since most botanical
worm medications do not affect the eggs, repeated treatments are
needed to ensure newly hatching larvae are cleared from the body.

Many herbs should never be used alone, because the most effective ones are very nasty and potentially toxic. Combinations of herbs
are required to prevent toxic side effects. Most over-the-counter
products are diluted to prevent these potential toxic effects, but their
effectiveness is also diluted. Some herbs are only safe in the proper
dosage, but may be highly toxic in excessive amounts. It is important
to evaluate the strength of the person as well as the parasite when
prescribing. How much and how often to take the product can mean
the difference between success and failure to treat parasites. Usually
the dosage on the label is for adults weighing approximately 150
pounds. Children, the elderly, or debilitated people should use less.
Most of these herbs are contraindicated in pregnancy and caution
should always be taken with children (see the guidelines for dosing
children). Parasite formulations with high quality ingredients, and
the proper combinations of herbs, will be tolerated much better.
This way a high level of the needed medicine can be prescribed with-

out a negative response. Getting the right ingredients, combinations and potency is the key, because some suppliers will sell just about anything.

Sometimes, a laxative herb is used in the formula to expel worms. Sometimes it is better to use a laxative separately. Laxatives are herbs that actively stimulate the bowels to promote movements. Stimulating laxatives should not be used long term. Their action occurs from 8-12 hours after taking. Some of these herbs cause griping pain in the abdomen, but look for those that are mild and gentle. They can be used safely and not present too many side effects. Do not use when intestinal cramps, bleeding sores, or hemorrhoids are present.

When it comes to herbal medications, you should only use the manufacturer's recommended dosage unless you are under the care of a trained health provider such as someone trained in herbal medicine, or a naturopathic physician. The following herbs have been historically used to help with parasitic infections.

ALLIUM SATIVUM (GARLIC)

Worldwide, people use garlic as a food, spice, and medicine to treat a number of infectious diseases. The active medicine, allicin, is released after the garlic cloves are minced, crushed, chewed, cut, or pressed. Allicin is responsible for the characteristic odor of garlic. Deodorized concentrates may contain only 30 to 100 parts per million of allicin and may be of questionable therapeutic value against parasites.

Garlic prevents and fights infection from different species of yeast, as well as fungus, bacteria, virus, and protozoa diseases. Garlic is also effective against roundworms, tapeworms, pinworms, and hookworms including: *Ascaris lumbricoides*, *Entamoeba histolytica*, *Giardia lamblia*, and *Trypanosoma* species. Garlic can cause dermatitis and irritation to the digestive tract. Some people are unable to effectively detoxify allicin and other sulfur-containing components. Generally, it is nontoxic to most individuals at the dosage commonly used.

ANGELICA ARCHANGELICA/SINENSIS

This herb, along with *Echinacea purpurea*, is one of the most widely used herbs for the treatment of the protozoa, *Trichomonas*. *Angelica* contains coumarin compounds that have been effective against this organism, as well as other worms and parasites. There are two commonly used species of *Angelica,* the Chinese variety, *Angelica sinensis* (dong quai) and the American and European species, *Angelica archangelica.* The two are not the same in their effects and the Chinese specie is superior as a treatment for all ailments of the female reproductive system. The Chinese herb relieves pain by reducing cramping in muscles, but may not be as effective in the treatment of *Trichomonas.* Pregnant women should not use this herb; neither should diabetics, as it tends to increase the sugar in the blood.

ARTEMISIA ABSINTHIUM (WORMWOOD)

Wormwood is one of the plants that settlers brought to America from Europe to treat worms. Even the ancients knew of its ability to kill parasites in the intestines and expel worms, especially roundworms, threadworms, and pinworms. It is still found in many parasite formulas on the market today and is used similarly to *Artemisia annua.* This specie of *Artemisia* is effective for worms such as *Ascaris lumbricoides* (giant intestinal roundworm) and *Enterobius vermicularis* (pinworm).

Wormwood is an intensely bitter herb that has found great favor with many herbalists as an agent against worms. This is because parasites are generally repelled or destroyed by herbs with strong bitter flavors. The dried and powdered flowers are excellent for expelling worms. The plant's leaves are sufficient to eliminate all live worms and many other parasites. Wormwood is more toxic when used alone. It is best combined with other herbs to nullify its toxicity. Avoid giving to children. The oil of wormwood is especially toxic at a minimum adult dose of 15 ml Some of the toxic symptoms are:

- Acute: headache, trembling, stupor, and convulsions
- Chronic: disturbed rest, disagreeable dreams, morning nausea and vomiting, epileptic attacks, physical and mental force impaired, impotence or premature menopause, restlessness, insomnia, nightmares, vomiting, vertigo, tremor, and convulsions

ARTEMISIA ANNUA (CHINESE WORMWOOD)

This traditional Chinese herb, also known as sweet wormwood, has been used in China for 2000 years. It is found in many parts of the world, but was not recognized until the early 1970s for its potential in treating the causative agent of malaria, *Plasmodium falciparum*. It is this particular herb that contains the chemical, artemesin, not found in any other species of *Artemesia*. It is reported to be the prototype for new antimalarial medicines.

This herb exerts a broad spectrum of activity against protozoa and yeast. It is effective against the liver fluke, *Clonorchis sinensis,* and the blood fluke, *Schistosoma japonicum,* as well as against giardia and other protozoa. This herb has a low toxicity level since no obvious side effects have been reported. It is safe in people with heart, kidney, or liver disease, and in pregnant women. Do use caution because Chinese wormwood can initially cause a worsening of symptoms, allergic reactions, and some intestinal irritation.

This herb is highly effective and quick acting. *Artemisia annua* crosses the blood-brain barrier making it potentially useful for the therapy of amebic infection in the brain. High dose antioxidant supplementation should be withheld during the treatment of protozoan infection, especially during treatment with *Artemisia annua.* When taking for cryptosporidium infection, use 1000 milligrams three times a day for 20 days. This herb may be given along with grapefruit seed extract or other antiparasitic herbs. When treating malaria with Artemisia annua, use for 10 days.

ARTEMISIA CINA (WORMWOOD, LEVENT WORMSEED)

This specie of *Artemisia* is very effective against worms, including pinworms, threadworms, and roundworms, especially the roundworm, *Ascaris lumbricoides*. Since this herb is very bitter, children usually take it with honey or in pill form, if possible. *Artemisia cina* combines well with *Cassia marilandica* (American senna). When treating *Ascaris lumbricoides*, it is important to dose correctly. Repeat treatment with this herb after one week.

This herb can be fatal in a dose of 1/2 ounce; less in a child. Use with caution, especially in pregnancy. Toxic symptoms include abdominal cramps, nausea and vomiting, coldness and pallor, headache, vertigo, diarrhea, profuse sweating, flushed face, foaming at the mouth, dilated pupils, twitching eyes and head, clenching of teeth, convulsions, cramps, and other central nervous system problems. In some cases the urine changes color from yellow saffron to reddish-purple.

BERBERINE-CONTAINING PLANTS

Berberine-containing plants have been used as an antibiotic and antiparasitic for 3000 years in traditional and folk medicine around the world. *Hydrastis canadensis* (goldenseal), *Berberis vulgaris* (barberry), *Berberis aquifolium* (Oregon grape), and *Coptis chinensis* (goldthread), share similar effects on parasites due to their high content of berberine. Berberine may not be as potent as many prescription antibiotics, but it will exhibits antimicrobial activity against protozoa and fungi including *Giardia lamblia, Entamoeba histolytica, Trichomonas vaginalis, Treponema pallidum, Leishmania donovani* (visceral leishmaniasis), and even many viruses and bacteria. Consider using berberine-containing plants in any infectious processes involving these organisms. It also inhibits the overgrowth of yeast that is a common side effect of antibiotic use. Berberine appears not to be harmful against non-pathogenic bowel flora such as the *Lactobacillus* species.

Berberine-containing plants has remarkable antidiarrhea activity even in the most severe cases, such as with *Giardia lamblia*. Experimental results indicate that these plants are particularly useful in diarrhea caused by the bacteria, *Escherichia coli*, and effective in treating the majority of common gastrointestinal infections. These properties have led to the production of berberine-containing products useful in the treatment of bacterial overgrowth, intestinal microflora imbalances, diarrhea, yeast overgrowth, protozoa infestations and increased intestinal permeability. Berberine also increases the blood supply to the spleen, improving the body's immune system and activates the white blood cells called macrophages.

The dosage of any berberine-containing herb should be based on the berberine content. Since there is a wide range of quality in the different products available, it is important to use standardized extracts. The therapeutic dose of berberine is typically 200 milligrams 2-3 times daily. The following is an example of a berberine containing formulation available for the treatment of parasites: *Berberis vulgaris* (barberry) 200 mg, *Berberis aquifolium* (Oregon grape) 200 mg, *Hydrastis canadensis* (goldenseal) 50 mg. During an acute infection, take 1-3 caps of the above formula three times a day.

The salt of berberine, berberine sulfate, has been used for centuries as an antimicrobial medication in China and India. It is widely distributed throughout nine plant families. Berberine sulfate exhibits antimicrobial activity against a wide variety of microorganisms, especially the digestive tract. Berberine sulfate can inhibit the growth of yeast, including *Candida albicans* and *Candida tropicalis*. Berberine also inhibits the growth of the protozoans *Entamoeba histolytica*, *Giardia lamblia*, *Trichomonas vaginalis*, and *Leishmania*. The effect of berberine sulfate increases with an increase in pH. At a pH of 8.0, its antimicrobial activity is typically 2-4 times greater than when it is at pH of 7.0 which is 1-4 times greater than a pH of 6.0. This suggests that alkalinization will improve its effect.

Children ranging from 5 months to 14 years of age were given berberine sulfate orally in a daily dose of 10 mg/kg/day for ten days. On the tenth day of treatment 90 percent of the berberine group had a negative stool culture for giardia. This compared to 95 percent for the prescription drug metronidazole (Flagyl). At a one month follow-up 83 percent of the berberine group continued to have a negative stool culture compared to 90 percent for the Flagyl group. Berberine sulfate is a safe and non-toxic treatment option for giardia, particularly in children. It should also be seriously considered in the management of *Trichimonas vaginalis*, both as an oral and topical treatment.

For those planning to travel to underdeveloped countries or areas of poor water quality or sanitation, the prophylactic use of berberine-containing botanicals one week prior to, during, and one week after the visit may be useful. The dose used is a single oral dose of 400 milligrams berberine sulfate. This would equate to a dose of approximately 4 grams of a goldenseal extract standardized to contain 8 percent berberine.

Berberine sulfate proved nontoxic and a satisfactory cure for giardia in children when given in an oral dose of 10 mg/kg/day for 10 days. A dose of berberine sulfate in mice of approximately 25 mg/kg did not produce gross toxic effects. Berberine sulfate and berberine-containing plants are generally considered to be non-toxic at recommended doses. High doses can result in the following side effects: lowered blood pressure, difficulty breathing, flu-like symptoms, gastrointestinal discomfort, and heart damage. Most berberine-containing plants are considered uterine stimulants, so care is cautioned during pregnancy.

BETULA LENTA (MOUNTAIN MAHOGANY, BIRCH)

The leaves and shoots are used as a laxative usually in combination with other herbs. Both the leaves and the bark have a bitter taste making it useful in the treatment of expelling worms. Children's dosage should be in proportion to age. There does not appear to be any overdose hazard, but it is possible to become poisoned on the methyl salicylate in the bark.

CALENDULA OFFICINALIS (CALENDULA)

Calendula used as an oil, or in a salve, or as a poultice, will stop bleeding, as well as soothe the pain and irritation and promote the healing of wounds. A tea made from one tablespoon of flowers to 1/4 quart of water is said to expel worms. Calendula promotes tissue repair and is well tolerated by most people.

CAPSICUM SPECIES (CAYENNE)

Cayenne can be added to a treatment plan to kill parasites. The dried ripe fruits contain the volatile oil capsaicin, recommended for digestive disorders. It has some analgesic effects similar to ginger. Cayenne does present a real danger if there is an existing ulcer or chronic irritation of the bowel. Bleeding and serious damage may occur in these cases. Excessive amounts can cause severe irritation of the digestive tract and may cause nausea, vomiting, and diarrhea.

CASCARA SAGRADA/RHAMNUS PURSHIANA (CASCARA)

Cascara helps with waste elimination by being a mild and effective laxative, especially in cases of chronic constipation. It is milder than Senna, with its main site of action being the lower bowel. This herb is safe in recommended dosage and found in many of the over-the-counter laxative preparations.

CASSIA ANGUSTIFOLIA AND CASSIA SENNA (SENNA)

Both the leaves and pods (fruits) were used in ancient Arab medicine as a safe and effective laxative. Today, senna is recognized as one of the most popular and reliable stimulant laxatives. The use of senna is generally regarded as safe. Since long-term dependence may develop, it is recommended only for short term use. Its chief action is on the lower bowel, causing mucus secretions and rapid contractions. It is best to combine senna with aromatic herbs for the digestive tract such as cardamom, ginger, and fennel, to reduce cramping. In proper dosage its action is mild, yet effective.

CEPHAELIS IPECACUANHA (IPECAC)

Ipecac has been successfully used to treat amebic dysentery. This herb will induce vomiting and cause the stomach to empty unless it is used in small quantities. In 1959, its analog, dehydroemetine, was introduced and found to be less toxic on the heart muscle.

CHENOPODIUM AMBROSIOIDES VAR. ANTHELMINTICUM (WORMSEED)

Wormseed was used for centuries by the Native Americans in combination with laxative herbs. This is a very bitter herb used for paralyzing roundworms, hookworms, and whipworms, with less effect upon tapeworms or threadworms. Then it takes a purgative or a laxative herb to move the parasite out of the body. Do not fast before using. Wait at least 2 weeks before repeating treatment.

Wormseed is very bitter and is usually preferred when given in capsule form. The little, glossy, black seeds would be the only safe use for home medicine. Otherwise, it should be noted that the plant is basically poisonous. The oil of wormwood is widely used against roundworms, hookworms, and intestinal ameba in tropical America, although the therapeutic dose is close to toxic levels. Death may result from such undesirable side effects from the central nervous system as convulsions, heart, and respiratory abnormalities. Do not use in heart, liver, kidney, stomach, or intestinal disease, or in pregnancy. Caution should always be used with children. A one-year-old baby died after receiving 4 drops three times a day for 2 days.

CUCURBITA PEPO (PUMPKIN SEED)

Pumpkin seeds are a traditional remedy for worms, being safe and somewhat effective against tapeworms, roundworm, threadworms, and pinworms, in both animals and humans. Seeds of several species of the genus, *Cucurbita,* have long enjoyed a considerable reputation as agents that paralyze and expel intestinal worms. The seeds of the autumn squash, *Cucurbita maxima,* and of the Canada pumpkin or crookneck squash, *Cucurbita moschata,* have similar properties.

The substance that affects the worms is quite variable even in seeds of the same species. This makes it very difficult to know how much it will take to get results. Although toxicity or undesirable side effects associated with pumpkin seeds have not been reported, their reliability varies too much to be useful. It does have the great advantage of being entirely safe. Use pumpkin seeds when more toxic herbs cannot be used, such as in pregnancy, ill people, liver disease, and children. It is important to take something to move the worms out of the digestive tract, because the pumpkin seeds merely paralyze the worm and does not kill it.

When you use the seeds, try to leave the fine inner skin beneath the shell intact, because it is important to eat this skin with the seeds. Keep to a healthy diet and take the seeds every morning on an empty stomach. Chew well. Children are given 10-15 seeds a day and adults 20-30 seeds for about two weeks. Take a purgative or laxative, one hour after each dose of seeds. An increased number of pumpkin seeds need to be eaten if tapeworms are the problem. You can repeat this treatment as often as necessary without any danger of side effects. With tapeworms make sure that the entire worm is expelled. Eating pumpkin seeds regularly may help to prevent these parasites.

CURCUMA LONGA (TURMERIC)

This is the root used to give the golden color to curry powder and to most Indian dishes. Turmeric has been used for generations in India to treat dysentery and expel worms from the body. This herb may be used as a blood purifier and can be applied internally and externally to heal wounds. Turmeric contains a substance that limits the inflammation caused by extensive tissue damage from parasites. Because turmeric may also stimulate the production of bile, it should be avoided when treating giardia. Bile stimulates giardia's growth and proliferation. There has not been any reported toxicity at standard doses, but high doses may damage the digestive system by causing ulcers.

DAUCUS CAROTA (WILD CARROT)

When treating for threadworms, do not serve anything but coarse or finely grated wild carrots for 1-2 days. During the worm's inactive state, juice the garden variety carrot and drink a glass each day or 1-2 large carrots for breakfast daily. Never fast a child without being under a physician care.

DRYOPTERIS FELIX-MAS OR ASPIDIUM FILIX-MAS (MALE FERN)

This plant has definite medicinal value recognized for centuries as deadly to intestinal worms such as flatworms and roundworms. Valuable medicinal properties include both plants, but *Aspidium filix-mas* is the primary herb of choice for the treatment of tapeworms. This herb paralyzes the voluntary muscles of the intestine as well as the contractile tissue of the tapeworm. Although it does not kill the parasite, the paralyzed worms are readily washed out of the bowels by an active purge. Sometimes, the tape worm does not passed out of the body intact, but gets dissolved and digested so that it is not possible to record success instantly. It will be apparent from the fact that no more worm sections are passed with the stools.

At the same time you take male fern, it is important to take dandelion root or silymarin extract to help protect the liver from the toxic effects of this plant. Caution is needed to avoid poisoning since it takes a large dose of eight to ten grams of the extract to kill the tapeworm. Symptoms can be produced even in therapeutic doses such as nausea, vomiting, cramping, and headache. If the dosage is too small, there will be failure to paralyze the parasite. If the dosage is excessive, it becomes an irritant poison causing muscular weakness, eyesight problems, liver damage, and possibly coma.

There should be caution used in people who already have liver damage or who have had jaundice due to virus hepatitis. People who are constipated need to have their bowels moving regularly before using this plant. Avoid in pregnancy, the elderly, and debilitated people, or people with ulcers, anemia, and kidney dysfunction. Do not take with fixed oils, fats, or alcohol because they increase absorption, thus increasing the toxicity. The powdered plant tends to lose its potency rapidly.

ECHINACEA PURPUREA (PURPLE CONEFLOWER)

Echinacea is useful for treating all chronic and acute bacterial and viral infections and parasites. It is one of the most widely used herbs for the treatment of *Trichomonas vaginalis*. Echinacea is an effective blood and lymphatic cleanser, and strengthens the immune system. It can be used internally and externally, apparently without toxic side effects and is effective in douches for the treatment of all vaginal infections.

EUGENIA CARYOPHYLLATA (CLOVES)

Traditional Indian Ayurvedic and Chinese healers used cloves to kill internal parasites. This spice exhibits a broad range of antimicrobial activity against other organisms, as well as fungi and bacteria. Cloves also help to increase the circulation of the blood, promote digestion, and eliminate gas and intestinal spasms. Cloves kills the eggs of parasites when taken orally.

FICUS GLABRATA (FICIN)

Ficus has been a well-known antiworm remedy in the tropical regions since ancient times. It is widely used by the natives of South America and the Panama region. The latex gathered from these trees has been commercially exploited for decades because of its enzyme properties containing papain and bromelain. The intestinal parasites commonly controlled by ficin include: *Ascaris lumbricoides* (giant intestinal roundworm), *Strongyloides stercoralis* (threadworm), *Trichuris trichiura* (whipworm), *Ancylostoma/Necator* (hookworm), *Taenia solium/saginata* (pork/beef tapeworm), *Enterobius vermicularis* (pinworm), and *Hymenolepsis nana* (dwarf tapeworm). It is the enzymes that digest the living worms, yet this plant is well tolerated and nontoxic to humans when taken internally. Even though the toxicity to ficin is low and it is not absorbed by the gastrointestinal tract, it is still not recommended during pregnancy.

FOENICULUM VULGARE (FENNEL SEED)

Fennel seeds help to remove waste material and parasites from the body. Fennel is generally used as a digestive aid and flavoring agent. This is not a dangerous plant, but the oil extracted from it can cause skin irritation, nausea, vomiting, seizures, and edema of the lungs. This plant should not be confused with several other common types of fennel, including dog fennel.

GENTIANA LUTEA (YELLOW GENTIAN)

The active ingredients of *Gentiana lutea* have been used historically for malaria. This gastric stimulant is used to improve digestion and treat all types of digestive disorders and has a strong activity against the protozoa, *Entamoeba histolytica*. It also expels intestinal worms and has antiseptic properties. Gentian strengthens the human system and is an excellent tonic to combine with a laxative herb, so that gentian is prevented from being toxic. Since it is a bitter herb, gentian is more palatable combined with an aromatic herb such as orange peel. This herb may not be tolerated well by those with very high blood pressure or by expectant mothers.

GRAPEFRUIT SEED EXTRACT

Research shows that grapefruit seed extract is effective against approximately 800 bacteria and virus strains, 100 strains of fungi, as well as a great number of single-cell parasites. No other known antimicrobial can make such claims. Despite inhibiting harmful intestinal parasites, when taken in a normal dose, grapefruit seed extract doesn't reduce the normal healthy bowel flora significantly.

Other countries have used grapefruit extract for the treatment of parasitic infections for some time. It has been used primarily throughout South America, Europe and the far east for its broad spectrum application as an antibiotic, antifungal, antiprotozoan, antiviral, antiseptic, disinfectant, and as a preservative in cosmetics. In South America it has long been used instead of chlorine in a variety of public swimming and bathing applications, as well as for sewage-water treatment. It can be used for treating drinking water since chlorinated water can damage sensitive intestinal flora. Chlorinated water does not kill various pathogenic organisms such as *Giardia lamblia*. In Peru, it is used for disinfecting agricultural products.

Dr. Louis Parish, M.D., as investigator for the Department of Health and Human Services, Public Health Service, Food and Drug Administration, reported that grapefruit seed extract is as effective as any other amebicide now available, perhaps more effective, and does not cause side effects. When traveling abroad, including Mexico or South America, grapefruit seed extract is an exceptional and simple alternative to the more harsh methods of killing parasites and other harmful organisms. Animals also seem to respond well to grapefruit seed extract. Pet owners report that it works as an effective natural alternative to chemical dewormers. The extract is usually available from health food stores.

For external use, never apply grapefruit seed extract full strength to the skin. The standard dilution is 33 percent grapefruit seed extract and 67 percent glycerin. For some application, it is best to dilute it with almond, olive, sesame or avocado oils, instead of water. Keep it away from the eyes, because of its ability to be irritating. Add a few drops of the extract to household cleaners, dishwashing soap or laundry detergents to ensure a germ-free environment in homes. This extract makes a great food wash for parasites and other pathogens.

Never use full strength when taking internally. Start with one drop dissolved in glycerin and then mixed with a glass of water or fruit juice, and slowly increase it according to your reaction. Work up to about 8 drops (or a corresponding number of capsules or tablets) in a full glass of water two to three times a day until symptoms disappear. When the organisms you are trying to kill begin to die, the toxins are released leading to discomfort or tiredness. If the symptoms are already too uncomfortable, reduce the amount of extract you are taking and begin increasing it very slowly when you feel more comfortable.

Since grapefruit seed extract can be very bitter, the debittered powder used in capsules may be a better choice. For children you can open a capsule and mix it in a glass of water or juice. In pill form it may take 100–300 milligrams daily to be effective for adults. Take one or two drops in a glass of water once or twice a day as a preventive for traveler's diarrhea or "Montezuma's revenge." This extract is nontoxic and friendly to the environment. Use caution if you are allergic or sensitive to citrus. Grapefruit seed extract is not absorbed into the intestinal tissue, is generally hypoallergenic, and can be taken safely up to several months. This amount of time may be required to eliminate giardia and yeast infections.

INULA HELENIUM (ELECAMPANE)

This herb can be of great benefit for lung ailments and digestive disorders, including weak digestion in the stomach and poor assimilation. The Chinese use it to counteract ingested poisons. Elecampane is specific for the roundworm, *Ascaris lumbricoides,* and recommended as the safest herb for children. It has a paralyzing effect on the worm's central nervous system.

JUGLANS CINEREA (BUTTERNUT)

This is a good general purpose herb for constipation or to get things moving and expel worms, especially threadworms and pinworms. Butternut can be safely combined with any other mixture for decreased bowel tone, to clean out the bowels, and as a soothing laxative in cases of chronic constipation. Do not take for a long time. A skin rash can occur when the juice of the leaves are used externally. When taken internally, butternut has caused some cases of nausea and vomiting.

JUGLANS NIGRA (BLACK WALNUT HULLS)

The black walnut hulls are known for their ability to kill many kinds of worms, especially tapeworms, in the digestive tract, but it is present only in the immature green hull surrounding the nut. This green hull must be harvested before the nut falls to the ground. The primary active constituent is known as juglone and exerts antifungal, antiworm, antiviral, antibacterial effects. An extract can be used safely in recommended doses by adults, but should be avoided by infants and small children.

LARREA DIVARICATA (CHAPARRAL)

Chaparral is one of the best herbal antibiotics, being useful against bacteria, viruses, and parasites, both internally and externally. It can be taken internally for the intestinal tract infections, diarrhea, and urinary tract infections. It is frequently combined with other antibiotic herbs such as goldenseal and echinacea. Externally, chaparral is applied to wounds as an antiseptic, to the skin for itching, and for eczema and scabies.

LINUM USITATISSIMUM (FLAXSEED)

Flax seeds comes from the same flax plant as does linseed oil. It is often given orally for its soothing action on the intestinal tract and as a source of bulk fiber. Overdoses have been reported because the plant does contain cyanide and nitrates. The immature seeds grown in warm climates are especially high in these toxins. Symptoms of an overdose could include an increased respiratory rate, excitement, gasping, staggering, weakness, paralysis, and convulsion. Skin reactions to flaxseed are fairly common. It might be best to limit your use of this plant substance or find another source of bulk fiber.

MELALEUCA ALTERNIFOLIA (TEA TREE OIL)

Tea tree oil is another powerful agent. A solution will be highly effective against *Trichomonas vaginalis* as a daily vaginal douche when using a 0.4 percent solution of melaleuca oil in one quart of water, twice a day, or one suppository at night. When used in this amount, it does not usually produce toxic symptoms.

MONARDA PUNCTATA (HORSEMINT)

Horsemint contains a large amount of thymol making it a powerful disinfecting agent. Almost 50 percent of this oil is excreted in the urine when taken internally, making it slightly useful as a urinary antiseptic. The primary uses have been for both external and internal worms, bacteria, and fungus. The mint has an aromatic odor and a warm, bitter taste. There have been no reports of toxic ingestion, but it can be irritating to the tissues. Rashes are common with external use. A significant amount of plant material would be needed to become toxic when taken internally.

OLEA EUROPEA (OLIVE LEAF EXTRACT)

The bitter substance in the leaf is the medicine produced by the olive tree, but eliminated from olives when they are cured. A new processing technique applied to an old herbal remedy has produced a nontoxic herbal parasite remedy. Olive leaf is effective against parasitic protozoa and other parasites, as well as fungi, molds, worms, and bacteria. It can also be used for yeast infections. For the last 4,000 years, populations in countries bordering the Mediterranean (Morocco, Italy, Sicily, Spain, France, Greece, Turkey, Israel, Egypt, Albania) have swallowed chopped up olive leaves in liquid or salad form to prevent or treat parasitic infections.

The olive leaf appears to have been a popular folk remedy superior to quinine for malarial infections, but was not as easy to administer, so quinine was preferred. Studies conducted during the late 1960s indicated that olive leaf extract has the ability to counteract the malaria protozoa. Supplements have become available and have a promising future against a wide variety of tropical diseases.

The method of how this product is manufactured is very important. Otherwise, the ingredients bind rapidly to serum proteins in the blood rendering them virtually useless in living organisms. The recommended dosage is four caps daily, taken throughout the day. If the "die-off" effect causes problems, the number of caps can be reduced to 3, 2, 1 or none, until the person feels better. A detoxification program may be recommended that includes vitamin C, along with supplements to ensure beneficial microflora in the bowel.

The "die-off" effects different people in different ways, usually depending on the extent of infection in the body. Individuals who have serious chronic fatigue syndrome or who harbor a large parasitic burden in their bodies may experience extreme fatigue, headaches, muscle or joint pain, or flu-like symptoms. These symptoms can begin almost immediately. Reduce the dosage or even stop medication until the symptoms stop, allowing the body to detoxify at a slower pace. Normally, olive leaf extract itself does not produce adverse side effects.

PLANTAGO PSYLLIUM (PSYLLIUM SEED HUSK)

Psyllium is a major source of fiber. The primary use of the seed or the seed husks is as a bulk laxative, especially for cases of chronic constipation. The tiny seeds contain a coating of gelatinous material that swells upon contact with moisture. One gram of seeds will swell to 8-14 times its volume when taken with water. A normal dosage ranges from 4-5 grams. This increases movement within the colon and produces a bowel movement, while cleansing the intestines and removing toxins. There have been no serious reports of toxicity with this plant. Do not use in people with bowel obstruction or bowel diseases without consulting your physician first.

PODOPHYLLUM PELTATUM (AMERICAN MANDRAKE, MAYAPPLE)

This herb is usually recommended for the treatment of constipation and sluggish bowel function. American Mandrake can be irritating to the intestinal membranes and toxic symptoms may occur from eating the green fruit or eating or handling the foliage or roots. Severe cases may result in drowsiness and lethargy. Do not confuse with the plant *Mandragora officanarum*, called mandrake by the Greeks and Asiatics.

PUNICA GRANATUM (POMEGRANATE)

The fruit rinds and bark are very astringent and are used to remove tapeworms and roundworms. The pomegranate roots had widespread use against tapeworm until less toxic substances were discovered. The plant contains an alkaloid that can be toxic if consumed in large quantities. Toxic symptoms could include muscle weakness, dizziness, vomiting, and diarrhea.

QUASSIA AMARA (PICRASMA EXCELSA)

The common Jamaica tree produces a bitter tonic useful for killing amebas, giardia, malaria, pinworms, and some roundworms such as *Ascaris lumbricoides*. The herb does not have a smell, but does have an intense bitter taste. This will distinguish the pure herb from adulterations. This herb contains a group of alkaloids known to inhibit protozoa from reproducing and effects their basic metabolic processes. Considerable evidence suggests that quassia is also effective against mosquito larva. Toxic symptoms are rare, but if they occur it is usually diarrhea, vomiting, or collapse. Large doses act as an irritant and cause vomiting. Quassia is also a nontoxic, inexpensive and effective treatment for head lice.

RHEUM RHAPONTICUM (RHUBARB ROOT)

Rhubarb acts as a laxative or mild purging agent. It combats some of the gripping associated with the herb, Senna, making it a useful in cases of dysentery and intestinal diseases. In small doses its astringency is used with diarrhea; larger amounts can cause severe diarrhea, cramping, and severe fluid loss. Safer and less drastic purgatives are available. This is not the common garden rhubarb, *Rheum rhaponticum*, which is not a strong purgative.

SALVIA OFFICINALIS (GARDEN SAGE)

The Romans recommended sage and thyme both as digestive aids and in the treatment of intestinal worms and bacteria. Sage was often mixed with wormseed or white wine to relieve diarrhea or dysentery. Garden sage is not highly toxic. Excessive amounts may cause dry mouth or local irritation.

SMILAX ORNATA (SARSAPARILLA)

Sarsaparilla root is useful as a blood purifier. This means that it cleanses and purifies the system. It is also used externally for the treatment of skin parasites. If the amount of toxins absorbed by the intestines are excessive, or if the liver is not filtering properly, the liver can become overwhelmed and allow toxins to circulate in the blood. Because the liver plays such a vital role in filtering toxic compounds absorbed from the intestinal tract, this herb can play a useful role in a formula for parasites. Evidence seems to support that this herb binds toxins.

SPIGELIA MARILANDICUS (PINKROOT)

Pinkroot is a highly effective vermicide, originally used by Native Americans. They introduced it to the settlers and early physicians.

The plant has the ability to cure infections from intestinal worms, especially roundworms and tapeworm, and some success with pinworms. It is even effective for the fevers caused by parasites. You can also give with a laxative such as *Cassia marilandic* (American senna) to decrease toxic symptoms. Pinkroot is a safe and efficient drug to give to children if administered in the proper lower doses. Large doses can produce side effects such as disturbed vision, dizziness, muscular spasms, twitching eyelids, increased action of the heart, plus frothing from the mouth, respiratory paralysis, and even convulsions.

TANACETUM VULGARIS (TANSY)

Tansy is largely used for expelling worms in children. For small children, reduce the dosage according to age. Care should be taken against overdoses. Fifteen drops of the oil, or 4 milliliters of the herb, could be fatal. Toxic symptoms include gastrointestinal irritation, nausea, vomiting, dizziness, headache, diarrhea, increased pulse rate, weak pulse, convulsions, paralysis, spasms, frothing from the mouth, respiratory paralysis.

THYMUS VULGARIS (THYME)

The Romans recommended sage and thyme both as digestive aids and in the treatment of intestinal worms. It is also antiseptic. It should not be used in large amounts, one ounce being adequate for a daily dose taken as tea. Externally, its antiseptic properties make it a useful mouthwash and cleansing wash for the skin. It will destroy fungal infections such as athlete's foot and skin parasites such as scabies, crabs and lice. For these purposes a tincture, or the essential oil, is used. When using thyme extracts containing essential oils internally, there is only a small margin of safety in its use.

TRIFOLIUM PRATENSE (RED CLOVER BLOSSOMS)

Red clover blossoms will kill flukes in all stages when used with cloves, black walnut hulls (green), and wormwood. The recommended dose is two capsules containing red clover blossoms three times daily. Red clover blossoms are themselves nontoxic, but other herbs used in the formulation can be toxic.

ULMUS FULRA (SLIPPERY ELM)

Take this herb internally for soothing and healing irritations of the intestinal tract. Make the powdered slippery elm into a gruel by gradually adding a small amount of water and mixing until the proper consistency is obtained. Sweeten the gruel with a little honey and a dash of cinnamon, cloves, and other spices for flavor. Slippery elm heals the stomach and intestinal ulcers very quickly. It also normalizes bowel function and relieves constipation and diarrhea, as well as being an excellent binder and cleanser. Externally, the moistened slippery elm can be applied to sores, wounds, and infected areas. Toxic ingestion has not been reported, but the plant may cause skin rashes when applied externally.

UNCARIA TOMENTOSA (CAT'S CLAW, UÑA DE GATO)

Cat's claw is a giant woody vine growing in the Peruvian tropical forests. It has properties that help in resistant cases of imbalanced intestinal flora, infection, sluggish digestion, poor assimilation, and bile stimulation. It is very effective as an intestinal cleanser and immune system rejuvenator, and possesses antimicrobial and anti-inflammatory activity. Cat's claw affects the ability of the white blood cells to engulf and digest harmful microorganisms. This is a good herb to accompany therapies for most parasites, but not giardia. The protozoa giardia actually thrives when there is bile stimulation. Cat's claw should not be used during pregnancy. It does seem to be quite safe for children, since it is virtually nontoxic.

ZINGIBER OFFICIANALIS (GINGER)

Ginger has worked against the roundworm, *Ascaris lumbricoides,* as well as the blood fluke, *Schistosoma mansoni,* and destroys the fish roundworm larvae of *Anisakis simplex.* Ginger also has been effective in the treatment of the dog heartworm, *Dirofilaria immitis.* There is evidence that ginger given in aqueous extracts from 2.5 percent up to 25 percent concentrations has been effective against the protozoa *Trichomonas vaginalis.* Ginger root is believed to have some analgesic effect and helps with inflammation similar to cayenne. It is used to treat nausea, vomiting, diarrhea, and stomach ache and has a long history of use for all types of digestive upsets, while also having antispasmodic effects. In general, the toxicity of this plant is low and its use in normally available amounts is not expected to produce toxicity.

CHAPTER 12

Holistic Treatments For Parasites

It is best not to treat yourself or your children without trained medical advice. Children have died from overdoses of medicine used to treat parasites. Sometimes, it can take laboratory testing before it is known whether or not the parasite is gone and the treatment has been completely effective. Unless all the worms and eggs are killed or expelled from the body, the infection will simply continue. The same goes for the many types of one-celled organisms that parasitize the human body. Only a physician can diagnose the presence of protozoans in a person. The person's stool or blood must be examined or an antibody test must be done.

Deworming treatments are not a solution for all intestinal parasites because protozoans and flukes are not affected by such medications. Solutions must be holistic and specific, and include education, proper sanitation and hygiene, and also adequate nutrition. Remember, many parasites do not manifest their presence by causing symptoms and therefore remain a reservoir of infection because the infected person does not seek treatment.

When considering how to use holistic approaches to ridding the body of a parasite, we must keep in mind that the human body is complex, elegant, and contains an efficient system of healing. Sometimes pharmaceutical drugs can interfere with this healing mechanism by suppressing the very symptoms that tell us what is going on in the body. Physicians who practice a holistic approach to healing use a variety of solutions for parasitic infection when possible. They use diet and nutrition, herbal medicine, homeopathy and other traditional medicines, as well as needed pharmaceutical drugs.

Not every case of diarrhea can be blamed on parasites. There are many bacteria that commonly cause intestinal distress. Unlike parasites such as giardia, bacteria generally run their course in a few days and do not recur at regular intervals. Keep track of any symptoms and write down the dates and times they occur. If you think you have parasites, ask your physician to give you a full stool-specimen test, as well as the other tests discussed in the chapter on laboratory analysis. If the doctor simply rules out giardia without trying either a stool or blood test, consider seeking out a physician that has training in parasites. If your doctor suggests that your symptoms are all in your head, it's time to find a new doctor.

The following is a quick review of what it usually takes to completely rid yourself of parasites:

1. Cleanse the intestinal tract.
2. Modify the diet.
3. Administer effective substances to eliminate parasites.
4. Recolonize the intestinal tract with friendly bacteria.
5. Eliminate risk factors to avoid reinfection.

Caution: When giving herbs or any remedy to infants or small children, only test small amounts. It is always best not to treat yourself or your children with many of the herbs and drugs used to kill or disable parasites. Always seek professional medical advice.

Digestive Enzymes

Eat foods that contain high amounts of digestive enzymes such as fresh pineapple and papaya. They contain bromelain and papain that break down the protein structures of parasites and aid to digest worms. Take 500 mg bromelain two to three times a day, especially for pinworms, along with a vegetarian diet. It is best to take bromelain and papain in their extract form so that you reduce this enzyme's sugar content. It may be necessary to add other digestive enzymes such as hydrochloric acid and pepsin.

Digestive enzymes may be needed to help digest and break down foods and promote better digestion and absorption of nutrients. Lifestyle factors such as chewing foods thoroughly are very important. This gives food adequate surface area for enzymatic activity to occur. Part of proper digestion is being relaxed when eating. Normal digestive secretions and motility do not easily happen if a person is anxious or depressed.

Enemas

Enemas are useful for cleansing the bowel and preparing the bowel to take an active role in ridding the body of toxic substances or infection. A hot water enema encourages blood flow to the abdomen. Intestinal parasites and other bowel problems can be treated with a hot enema. The unwise use of enemas in children can result in bowel perforation and rupture. People with chronic constipation or congenital diseases are especially likely to absorb large amounts of water from enemas, resulting in elevated hydrostatic pressure from the enema, which causes the perforation. If you select water for the enema use plain hot water at 104 to 110° F. Most herbal teas can be used at double strength as a cleansing enema. See the many ways enemas can be prepared for the treatment of worms in other sections of this chapter.

Essential Oils

The diverse antimicrobial action of essential oils has the ability to kill many types of worms, as well as the protozoa *Trichomonas vaginalis*. The essential oils of *Mentha piperita* (peppermint), and *Lavandula angustifolia* (lavender) has the fastest killing effects of 20 minutes and 15 minutes, respectively. The essential oil thymol is specific for hookworm. Caution should be used when using essential oils to treat parasitic infection. Many of them are toxic especially in children and people with heart, liver, kidney, stomach, or intestinal disease, as well as in pregnancy. Treatment with essential oils should not be done in anyone under the age of six.

Foods When Traveling

Select your food with care. Any raw food could be contaminated, particularly in areas of poor sanitation. Foods of particular concern include salads, uncooked vegetables and fruit, unpasteurized milk and milk products, raw meat, and shellfish. If you peel fruit yourself, it is generally safe. Food that has been cooked and is still hot is generally safe. For infants less than 6 months of age, breastfeed or give powdered commercial formula prepared with boiled water.

Some fish are not guaranteed to be safe, even when cooked, because of the presence of toxins in their flesh. Tropical reef fish, red snapper, amberjack, grouper, and sea bass can occasionally be toxic at unpredictable times if they are caught on tropical reefs rather than open ocean. The barracuda and puffer fish are often toxic, and should generally not be eaten. Highest risk areas include the islands of the West Indies and the tropical Pacific and Indian Oceans.

Foods That Parasites Don't Like

A consistently poor diet promotes very poor intestinal health, creating the perfect environment for parasites to live and grow. The diet with the highest resistance to worm infestation is high in unrefined carbohydrates, raw green vegetables, and adequate protein, and low in meat, pork, uncooked fish, and sugar. A good diet increases immune function, thereby protecting a person from infestation in the first place. Attention to the diet is essential with a reduction in all products containing white flour and other acid-forming foods so that the bowel contents become more alkaline. Read more about acid and alkaline foods in the chapter "Diet and Digestion." The ailments may not necessarily be cured by the following foods and suggestions, but may at least be alleviated. The following foods are naturally antiparasitic.

- To make a pumpkin seed infusion, steep 1 ounce crushed seeds for 15 minutes in 2 cups boiling hot water. Drink 1 tea cup to 1 pint daily for 1 to 3 weeks. You can also eat the seeds raw. You can also take pumpkin and watermelon seeds and grind them into a powder and them take with aloe vera juice on an empty stomach every morning. See the chapter "Medicinal Herbs" for more information about using pumpkin seeds.
- Pomegranates: eat 1–3 per day when in season.
- Fresh papaya seeds: 1 teaspoon to 1 tablespoon chewed daily on an empty stomach for a week. Stop for 2 days, then repeat for another week.
- At least 50 percent of your diet should be in the form of raw foods, especially lettuce, cabbage, and other salad greens.
- It is important to change the intestinal environment by changing

the diet. Worms love sugar, acid conditions, and constipation. High fiber, alkaline diets are the best prevention and cure.

- Avoid dairy products.
- Eat raw carrot salads with large amounts of fresh garlic.
- Use cayenne pepper.
- Eat 3–4 cloves of garlic a day for 1 week. Garlic is one of the most effective of the body cleansers. For a worm cure, roll dried garlic into pills or put garlic in salads. Eat a garlic bud first thing in the morning on an empty stomach.
- Fresh horseradish can be effective against some worms.
- Make lemon water with fresh, unstrained, and pitted lemons. It is cleansing for the system and will help eliminate worms in children. You can crush lemon seeds and take for five days. Stop for two weeks and repeat taking the seeds for two more weeks.
- Eat the sprigs of thyme freely. Use dried thyme in a sandwich, use thyme in pill form, or drink 1/2 cup of thyme tea each morning and evening to attempt to cleanse the system of worms.
- Rose hips made into a tea help to expel roundworms from the system.
- Bitter melon eaten as a vegetable is very effective in killing parasites.
- Eat tomatoes with ground black pepper.
- On an empty stomach in the morning eat 100 raw pumpkin seeds, then fast 5 hours and follow with fresh carrot juice. Repeat the next day if necessary.
- Take the white part of green onions and make into juice. Add 1-2 teaspoons sesame seed oil and take twice a day on an empty stomach for 3 days.
- Eat sunflower seeds every morning on an empty stomach.
- Drink the juice of one fresh coconut or eat 4 ounces of the flesh in the morning on an empty stomach. Then do not eat for 4 hours. Do this every day for a week if you have tapeworms.

Intestinal pH

Parasites prefer a digestive system that is too acidic. Most Americans eat a diet that is high in acid foods. It is important to begin balancing your diet with foods that are alkaline. See the chapter "Diet and Digestion" for more information on this subject.

Laxatives

It is very important to have proper bowel movements or the parasites recover from the treatment. One way to take a laxative is to drink aloe vera juice or to make a tea from senna leaves. See the chapter "Medicinal Herbs" for the listing of additional herbs used as laxatives.

Probiotics

The human body supports many life forms, both externally and internally. Most of these do little harm. Others can be beneficial such as the bacteria that colonize the intestinal tract. A healthy intestinal tract is loaded with friendly bacteria. These bacteria actually protect the body from the invasion of other more harmful viruses, bacteria, and parasites. Parasites can be fought with high dosages of probiotic substances such as *Lactobacillus acidophilus, bifidobacteria,* and *Lactobacillus bulgaricus.* Treatment needs to last for several months. The health and number of organisms making up the normal bowel flora needs to be strong in order to compete against potential pathogens. Intestinal parasites or yeast infections ravage the intestinal flora making it especially important to rebuild this bowel microflora after treating parasites. Increasing your probiotics is important in fighting off any further infestations.

Friendly bowel bacteria are often killed after taking antibiotics, since they kill the good as well as the bad bacteria. Without the help of these friendly bacteria, we would not manufacture the B vitamins. Also, foods with preservatives would not be broken down adequately for complete utilization. This puts too much strain on our friendly bacteria and many of them die. When they die, it is likely something else will take their place. But the replacement may not be so friendly.

Traveler's Diarrhea

- The best way to prevent traveler's diarrhea is by paying meticulous attention to your choices of food and drinks. Pepto-Bismol (2 ounces 4 times daily, or 2 tablets 4 times daily) appears to be an effective preventive agent, but is not recommended for prevention of traveler's diarrhea for more than a three-week period. It can be taken every 30 minutes for eight doses. Limit treatment to 48 hours at most, with no more than 8 doses in a 24-hour period. This preparation decreases the rate of diarrhea and usually shortens the duration of illness. Side effects of using Pepto-Bismol include temporary blackening of tongue and stools, occasional nausea and constipation, and rarely, ringing in the ears. This product should be avoided by people with aspirin-allergy, renal insufficiency, gout, and by those who are taking the anticoagulants, probenecid, or methotrexate. It is important for the traveler to consult a physician about the use of the bismuth subsalicylate found in Pepto-Bismol, especially in children, adolescents, and during pregnancy.

- Antidiarrheals such as Immodium can decrease the number of diarrheal stools, but can cause complication for persons with serious infections. These drugs should not be used by anyone with a high fever or blood in their stools. If you do become ill with traveler's diarrhea, it is usually self-limited and treatment requires only simple replacement of fluids and salts lost in diarrheal stools. This is best achieved by use of an oral rehydration solution such as World Health Organization Oral Rehydration Salts (ORS) solution. ORS packets are available at stores or pharmacies in almost all developing countries. ORS is prepared by adding one packet to boiled or treated water. Packet instructions should be checked carefully to ensure that the salts are added to the correct volume of water. ORS solution should be consumed or discarded within 12 hours if held at room temperature, or 24 hours if refrigerated.

- It is important for the traveler to consult a physician about treatment of diarrhea in children and infants, because some of the drugs and herbs mentioned are not recommended for them. The greatest risk for children is dehydration. Dehydration is best prevented by using the ORS solution in addition to the infant's usual food. The dehydrated child will drink ORS avidly; ORS is given ad lib to the child as long as the dehydration persists. The infant who vomits the ORS will usually keep it down if the ORS is offered by spoon in frequent small sips.

- Breast-fed infants should continue nursing on demand. For bottle-fed infants, give full-strength lactose-free, or lactose-reduced formulas. Older children receiving semi-solid or solid foods should continue to receive their usual diet during diarrhea. Immediate medical attention is required for the infant with diarrhea who develops signs of moderate to severe dehydration, bloody diarrhea, fever in excess of 102° F, or persistent vomiting. While medical attention is being obtained, the infant should be offered ORS.

• Most episodes of traveler's diarrhea resolve in a few days. As with all diseases it is best to consult a physician rather than attempt self-medication, especially for pregnant women and children. Travelers should seek medical help if diarrhea is severe, bloody, or does not resolve within a few days, or if it is accompanied by fever and chills, or if the traveler is unable to keep fluid intake up and becomes dehydrated.

• Consider taking along Pepto-Bismol as a diarrhea preventive. Take two ounces four times daily or one daily or one to two tablets four times a day for every day of travel. Freeze-dried acidophilus is a beneficial intestinal microflora that can help prevent traveler's diarrhea. Take on an empty stomach one-half hour before eating.

Water

• In areas with poor sanitation only the following beverages may be safe to drink: boiled water, hot beverages such as coffee or tea made with boiled water, canned or bottled carbonated beverages, beer, and wine. Ice may be made from unsafe water and should be avoided. It is safer to drink from a can or bottle than to drink from a container that is not known to be clean. However, water on the surface of a beverage can or bottle may also be contaminated. Therefore, the area of a can or bottle that will touch the mouth should be wiped clean and dry. Where water is contaminated, travelers should not brush their teeth with the local tap water.

Boiling is the most reliable method to make water safe to drink. Bring water to a vigorous boil, then allow it to cool; do not add ice. At high altitudes allow water to boil vigorously for a few minutes or use chemical disinfectants. Adding a pinch of salt or pouring water from one container to another will improve the taste. See the section "Medicinal Herbs" for information about grapefruit seed extract's use in disinfecting water.

If you are in doubt about the safety of your drinking water, then buy distilled water. As a last resort, if no source of safe drinking water is available, tap water that is uncomfortably hot to touch may be safer than cold tap water. However, many disease-causing organisms can survive the usual temperature reached by the hot water in overseas hotels. Boiling or proper disinfection is still advised. Dairy products can aggravate diarrhea in some people and should be avoided.

Other Holistic Therapies

- Bentonite clay found in most health food stores is a good natural parasite preventive. Take at least 1 tablespoon in the morning and evening. It has been reported that bentonite clay prevents travelers from parasites by absorbing poisons in the intestinal tract and flushing them out of the body.
- Diatomaceous Earth: Farmers have been using diatomaceous earth for years to prevent parasitic infestation with their farm animals. They simply mix this natural mineral-laden soft rock phosphate with the animal's meal and the intestinal problem treats itself. The diatomaceous earth acts like ground glass and cuts the segments and eggs that are released, as well as damaging the worm itself, causing it to let go. Mix four parts ground psyllium seed to one part diatomaceous earth. Take one rounded teaspoon every day for rebuilding and worm destroying. Children should take one-half the adult dosage.

Treatments for Protozoans

- In general, amebas are kept under control in India with jasmine tea, a semi-fermented black tea called "oolong" that contains jasmine flowers.
- Take 2 teaspoons liquid chlorophyll in 4 ounces water twice a day.
- Bitter melon eaten as a vegetable is very effective in killing protozoa.

The following suggestions are specific for each type of protozoa:

Cryptosporidium
- Try a homeopathic combination that incudes low doses of Cuprum, Ipecac, and protozoa. This combination is effective in wiping out cryptosporidium.
- DHEA fights crytosporidium. Ten elderly hamsters received DHEA prior to being inoculated with cryptosporidium. An additional ten hamsters were infected, but did not receive DHEA. Animals receiving DHEA had a significant reduction in the sever-

ity of cryptosporidium infection. DHEA is an immune modulator that has been shown to stimulate immune function. DHEA levels are frequently low in people with compromise immune systems. If this study can be applied to humans, then DHEA might be of value in the treatment of this organism. DHEA should only be prescribed by your physician.

Entamoeba histolytica
- Grapefruit seed extract gave symptomatic relief more than any other treatment.

Giardia
- Transfer factor (see the chapter "The Immune System's Role")
- Use one clove garlic with some added olive oil, applied to whole grain bread before meals; eat twice a day every five days; rest three days; repeat. Prepare the oil by peeling fresh garlic (4–8 oz.), mince, and put into a wide-mouth jar. Pour cold-pressed olive oil over it until all the garlic is covered. Tightly close and allow to set for up to seven days while shaking it daily. Strain and put in a dark bottle. Store in a cool place.
- A high fiber diet decreases giardia infections. Be sure to take adequate water when increasing fiber. Increase fiber intake slowly.
- Take digestive enzymes if needed.
- Grapefruit seed extract gives symptomatic relief more than any other treatment.

Toxoplasma gondii
- An ethanol extract of propolis has shown to be 100 percent lethal to the protozoan *Toxoplasma gondii* after 24 hours of contact. This extract will also decrease the inflammation associated with *Trichomonas*. Propolis is an amazing natural antibiotic found in leaf buds or the bark of poplars, chestnuts, and other common trees. Bees collect propolis, treat it with their own enzymes and use the sticky material to patch holes or cracks in their beehives. It actually creates an antibiotic disease-fighting reaction to almost any illness. It also stimulates the thymus gland and enhances the body's immune system. Inflammatory diseases have been treated successfully with propolis.
- Place two drops of the oil of sassafras on the soles of the feet twice daily.

Trichomonas vaginalis

- Betadine (Povidone-Iodine): It has a broad therapeutic effect in killing a large number of different microorganisms causing vaginitis, including *Trichomonas vaginalis*. Povidone-iodine has several advantages over iodine in that it has little sensitizing potential, does not sting, is water soluble, and washes out of clothing. It has been reported to have a success rate of 98 percent with a two week treatment regime using Betadine preparations. The usual treatment is using a betadine douche or saturated tampon twice a day for 14 days. Use 2 tablespoons or a 2.5 fluid ounces packet to one quart of lukewarm water. Other authors suggest a 28 day course. Avoid excessive use because some of the iodine will be absorbed into the body and possibly cause suppression of thyroid function.

- An ethanol extract of propolis has shown to be 100 percent lethal on the protozoan *Trichomonas vaginalis* after 24 hours of contact. This extract will also decrease the inflammation associated with *Trichomonas*. See the section above, *Toxoplasma gondii*, for more information.

- *Melaleuca alternifolia* (tea tree) oil is effective when used as a daily vaginal douch. Use a 0.4 percent solution of *Melaleuca* oil in one quart of water. Use one suppository at night. No adverse reactions have been reported and most people find *Melaleuca* soothing.

- Use lactobacillus culture yogurt douches daily, preferably in the morning. Do read labels carefully since most commercially available yogurts do not use lactobacilli. It is easier to insert one capsule of lactobacillus into the vagina twice daily for several weeks. *Lactobacillus acidophilus* is a desirable bacteria of the normal vaginal flora. It helps to maintain a healthy vaginal ecology by preventing the overgrowth of less desirable species.

- Keep the vaginal area acid. *Trichomonas* grows rapidly when conditions of the pH are between 5.5 and 5.8, such as with increased progesterone levels.

- Calcium and magnesium are important for certain pathways that may prevent *Trichomonas vaginalis*.

- Zinc supplements are important in the treatment of *Trichomonas* infections of both men and women. This suggests that persistent *Trichomonas* infections in men may be due to a low level zinc deficiency. Zinc sulphate at 220 mg twice a day for 3 weeks has been recommended as a possible treatment for this infection. Douche with one tablespoon of 2 percent solution in one pint water twice a day.

Plasmodium falciparum

- A supplemental treatment for this malaria-causing ameba consists of taking the temperature every 15 minutes and at the first sign of an elevation of body temperature, putting the person into a Russian steam bath, a whirlpool, or a hot bathtub, to elevate the temperature to about 102-103° F. This brings out white blood cells into the bloodstream to attack the parasites before they can enter a new red blood cell. This method will not get all of the malaria parasites, but will at least reduce the number. Be ready with a repeat of this method every time the temperature elevates and symptoms appear. Used with persistence and proper timing this treatment will reduce the numbers of organisms.
- You might consider taking 40-100 mg. of vitamin B1 per day. Or, you could take brewer's yeast tablets; take at least three tablets three times per day to help naturally repel both fleas and mosquitoes from your body.

Treatments for Worms

- The basis of all naturopathic philosophy centers on rebalancing the gastrointestinal tract. Due to incorrect nutritional habits, many people upset the acid/alkaline balance in their body. The balance is also disturbed by antibiotics and other drugs. Correct the imbalances and the worms disappear and do not likely reappear. Just don't give the worms a suitable environment to live and grow.
- Most worms are active during the full-moon cycle so it is easiest to treat them during this time. Start taking the herbs five days before the full moon and continue until you finish the treatment. The gestation period for the female worm is about 22 days. This means thousands of newborn worms every 22 days, plus all their waste products. This adds up. That is why you should not miss one day of any treatment plan. Many treatments last for anywhere from 30 days to three months.
- Take apple cider vinegar, 1-2 teaspoons in a glass of water.
- A garlic suppository can be affective against worms in the lower intestinal tract. Be careful not to nick the garlic when you peel it.
- Chop 1 clove garlic and place in a spoon. Fill the spoon the rest of the way with olive or sesame oil and swallow. Do not eat or drink until bowels have moved. Repeat the next day.
- Worms do not like the effect of pomegranates.

- Eat unsweetened pineapple juice.
- Drink peppermint tea.
- Crush fresh garlic and cover with olive oil 1-2 inches above the garlic. Steep 2 days, press out the oil, and eat 1 teaspoon on a piece of whole grain bread before or between meals. Eat twice a day for 5 days. Rest 3 days and repeat for 5 more days. Increase water and use a laxative.
- The raw juice of sauerkraut is effective in expelling worms, as is eating horseradish and onions.
- Eat nothing but 3-5 ounces of pumpkin seeds, plus 3-8 cloves of raw garlic per day.
- Take 500 mg of bromelain and 500-1000 mg of papain 3 times daily on an empty stomach.
- It may be necessary to take the digestive enzyme pancreatin (8X) in doses of 500 mg.
- Take 1 teaspoon of fig powder for its laxative effect.

Pinworms (Enterobius vermicularis)

- As with other infections, pinworms develop best when vitality is low. The biggest difference between people who get these worms and those that don't is diet. Those who are most susceptible are more likely to eat more refined carbohydrates and sugar and have much less fiber in their diet.
- Raisins soaked in senna tea for older children is a favorite remedy.
- Take the digestive enzyme bromelain in 500 mg doses 2-3 times a day.
- Bitter melon, a cucumber-shaped vegetable found in Chinese, Japanese, and Korean markets, is especially effective against pinworms. Eat in small pieces with other vegetables because of its bitter taste. It is recommended to eat one or two bitter melons a day for seven to ten days. Repeat after one to three months to make sure the infestation has not returned. If there are pinworms you will see many little white "bugs" in your stool the day after eating bitter melon. Bitter melon is a safe vegetable to eat.
- One of the best treatments is the use of a garlic enema. Place two cloves of garlic in a quart of water. Boil the water for a few minutes, then cool the liquid and place in an enema bag. Bring a chair to the edge of the bathtub and lie face down on the chair with legs hanging into the tub. Lubricate the anal opening, slide the enema tube in about an inch. Let the fluid run in and then out into the

tub. Repeat once a week. Drink a worm tea at the same time to stimulate bowel function, pushing the worms from the upper to the lower parts of the intestine and are finally expelled from the body.

- Another way to prepare a garlic enema is to take 2 cloves of garlic and mash them thoroughly, boil in 6 ounces of milk, let cool and strain. Prepare an enema, inject 4 ounces of this milk into rectum. Do this 3 nights in a row. Wait 7 days and repeat.
- A clove of garlic can be coated with olive oil and inserted directly into the rectum each evening.
- To relieve any itching in the rectum, an injection of warm water in which garlic or onions have been crushed will be beneficial. The outside of the rectum should be kept clean by washing with soap and water. As worms are inclined to migrate to the sexual organs. Itching in these parts may indicate their presence. The injection mentioned above should be used in these areas as well.
- Eat a garlic clove three or four times a day, or blend with olive oil and take in tablespoon doses. Eat as much as you can stand of the fresh garlic.
- Use a combination of one clove garlic, with some added olive oil, on whole grain bread before meals; take twice a day every 5 days; rest 3 days; repeat. Prepare the oil by peeling fresh garlic (4-8 oz.), mince, and put into a wide-mouth jar. Pour cold-pressed olive oil over it until all the garlic is covered. Tightly close and allow to set for up to 7 days while shaking it daily. Strain and put in a dark bottle. Store in a cool place.
- When using a tincture of garlic, take up to 25 drops in water several times a day as needed.

Roundworms (Ascaris lumbriocoides)

- Eat raw carrots and beets. Chew well and wash down with raw sauerkraut juice.
- Another good way of getting rid of roundworms quickly is to boil some garlic, horseradish and onions in water and drink it as hot as possible, but slowly, one sip at a time.
- Eat as much garlic as you can stand, then 2 days later take a laxative. Sit in a milk bath sufficient for covering the rectal area. Worms "smell" the milk and crawl out. Remain in the warm bath for about 1 hour until all the worms are out.
- Extracts of garlic, onion, pomegranate rind, turmeric (*Curcuma*

longa), and various citrus rinds possess anti-worm properties against *Ascaris*.

- Bromelain and papain and other proteolytic enzyme complexes are useful in dissolving the outer layer of the worms.
- Fig powder is useful for its laxative effect.

Hookworms (Ancylostoma duodenale/ Necator americanus)

- Treat anemia, which can caused by hookworm infection.
- It is important to wear shoes of some kind when in areas where hookworms are prevalent. Waking barefoot puts you at risk of hookworm infection.
- Drink 2 cups of strong thyme tea, followed by a dose of epsom salt one-half hour later.
- The essential oil thymol is specific for hookworm. Use caution when using essential oils, especially internally. Do not use with children.

Tapeworms

- Don't fast for long periods because tapeworms cannot be starved. It will only makes you feel weak and nauseated. When you finally take the medicine on an empty stomach, you may throw up. It is better to eat foods that the tapeworm doesn't like for a day or two. Eat foods such as onions, garlic, pickles and salted fish. This weakens the worm so they loosen their grip. Then they are easily dislodged.
- Treat for anemia because tapeworms can use up all the available vitamin B12 and cause pernicious anemia.
- Use a combination of one clove garlic, with some added olive oil, on whole grain bread before meals; take twice a day every 5 days; rest 3 days; repeat. Prepare the oil by peeling fresh garlic (4-8 oz.), mince, and put into a wide-mouth jar. Pour cold-pressed olive oil over it until all the garlic is covered. Tightly close and allow to set for up to 7 days while shaking it daily. Strain and put in a dark bottle. Store in a cool place.
- To help with all types of tapeworms try pumpkin seeds, cayenne, pine needles, and thyme. Start taking five days before the full moon. Make a tea and drink three 8-oz. cups a day.
- Eat a vegetarian diet and avoid all meat while continuing treatment.

ADDITIONAL NUTRITIONAL SUPPLEMENTS

- Take 500-1000 mg ascorbic acid or vitamin C three times a day.
- Take 20-50 mg of B-complex vitamin daily.
- Take chlorophyll to help with digestion and in cleansing the blood.
- Vitamin A is essential to decrease susceptibility to infectious organisms. Vitamin A is toxic in high dosages, so use caution in treating pregnant women, children, and the elderly. Take 25,000 IU a day of vitamin A or take 200,000 IU a day of beta carotene.
- Take 200-800 IU of vitamin E a day. Start at the lower dose and gradually increase the dosage.
- Iron deficiency can lower immune function. Too much iron can increase availability to microorganisms, leading to an increase in growth of the pathogen.

HOMEOPATHIC REMEDIES FOR PARASITES

Using homeopathic remedies allows your immune system to be gently and gradually enhanced. These remedies should not produce any harmful side effects and do not produce drowsiness or a medicated feeling. This is an advantage when treating children. Homeopathic formulas offer a combination of symptomatic relief without the side effects of prescription drugs.

Parasite treatment can be very complicated and should be supervised by a professional health care expert. Since homeopathic medications must be prescribed correctly before they will work, you may need to consult a health practitioner trained in homeopathy that can provide you with the correct remedy or remedies, especially for serious or chronic infections. To find a qualified physician in your area see your phone book yellow pages or contact the American Association of Naturopathic Physicians for more information (see "Resources" section at the end of book).

You will still need the addition of herbal medicine or other types of medication. You will probably need one type of treatment to kill the pathogen and a homeopathic remedy to modify the body's terrain and prevent the parasite form coming back. Usually homeopathic remedies do not kill the parasites. Instead, they make the environment that the parasites live in less "comfortable."

The person's mouth should be clean, meaning free of food and beverages. Avoid garlic and other strong odors, strong drinks, tobacco, smoke, toothpaste, mouthwash, gum, mints, or other foods and drinks at least 15 minutes before and after taking the homeopathic medication. Substances with strong odors can neutralize the action of the homeopathic remedy.

For symptoms caused by parasites, your doctor may prescribe adults 2–3 pellets of one of the following remedies three times a day. Liquids are given 10-15 drops under the tongue 3-4 times daily. In children, use half amounts and in infants quarter amounts. When symptoms are acute, it may be necessary to take the drops more than three times a day; sometimes as often as every 15 minutes to one-half hour. The best dosages for home use are 6X-6C or 30X-30C, unless stated otherwise.

It may be necessary to use remedies for the liver, blood and lymphatic system as well to rid the body of the toxins resulting from parasitic infection. Each of the following sections lists a number of homeopathic remedies, along with the symptoms specific to each parasitic condition.

Infection by Ameba
- Arsensicum 6C: Burning fever, great weakness and prostration, fluid retention, thirsty for sips of water, fatigue after passing diarrheal stool
- China 6C: Thirst before or after acute phase but not during it, chilliness not helped by warmth, sweating and weakness, attack preceded by restlessness and pains in joints
- China sulph 6C: Chills, fever and sweating, thirst, pains in spine
- Cinchona officinalis 9C: Painless diarrhea, painful diarrhea relieved by bending forward, lingering effects of malaria
- Sulphur 6C: If none of the remedies above seem suitable, take homeopathic sulphur

Infection by Worms
- Artemesis vulgaris 6C: Epileptic and convulsive states, sleep walking, brain congestion
- Baryta carbonicum 6C: Crawling sensation in rectum, constipation, abdomen is hard and tense with intense colic, good for the roundworm *Ascaris lumbriocoides*
- Bell 30C: Wakes screaming, cannot be pacified, wets bed, eyes brilliant, skin dry, hot, violent rage when spoken to; cheeks are scarlet but other parts of the face, especially around mouth, are white
- Calcaria 12C: When child is fat, pale, with lymphatic congestion, head hot and perspiring at night, the perspiration not being offensive, feet cold and clammy

- Cina abrotanum 6-9C: Intestinal irritation, worm infestation, grinding teeth, jerking of hands and feet when relaxing, pulsation in upper eyeball area, picks nose, rings around eyes, hungry, itching of anus, very cross and irritable, nervousness caused by worms, itching of the nose, fever, pale urine, wants to be rocked, skin sensitive to touch; works well on *Ascaris* lumbriocoides and other roundworms and tapeworms; this is a children's remedy especially if they are big, fat, rosy, with worms and accompanying complaints
- Cinchona 6C: Darting pains across abdomen, increased flatus and bitter eructation, pains in liver area, liver swollen, abdomen distended
- Ferrum mur 3C: anemia, passage of blood and mucus
- Filix mas 6C: Bloated, worse eating sweets, diarrhea and vomiting, worm colic, itching nose, blue rings around eyes, constipation, pale face, gnawing pain; primarily for tapeworms; generally not recommended for children
- Granatum 6C: Primarily for tapeworms; pain worse around umbilicus, itching about anus, constant hunger
- Graphites 6C: Fetid, sour stool; itching in the anal area, chronic diarrhea
- Lycopodium 12C: Distention of abdomen, poor appetite, constipation, dark thick urine, pains in the body going from right to left
- Mercurius corrosivus 6C: Rectal spasms, pain behind eyeballs, iritis, burning eyelids, nasal rawness and swelling, inflamed throat, dysentery, stool hot bloody slimy and offensive, great hunger, itching rectum, weakness, offensive breath, evacuations very painful, much mucus in the stool, distention of the abdomen, excessive saliva
- Naphthaline 6C: For worms, especially pinworms
- Natrum phosphoricum 6C: Especially for pinworms; picking at the nose and tendency to rheumatism
- Santoninum 3-6C: It is of unquestioned value in the treatment of worm diseases especially roundworms, with gastrointestinal irritations, itching of nose and anus, restless sleep, twitching of muscles
- Scirrhinum 6C: It has been observed the when prescribing a course of Scirrhinum and other cancer nosodes for people this was often followed by the expulsion of worms; intestinal parasites may be one symptom of the cancerous diagnosis. It also suggests that giving Scirrhinum 30C, once or twice a week should be included

among the remedies given for worms. An occasional dose of Scirrhinum 200C will often drive them away

- Sinapsis nigra 6C: This remedy is primarily for pinworms if Teucrium Marum Verum fails
- Spigelia marilandica 9C: Abdominal pains caused by worms, feeble, precocious children; feverish, dry, hot skin; furred tongue, nervous irritability, swollen abdomen, constipation, blue rings around the eyes, faint nauseated feeling with colic around the navel area, itching and crawling sensation in the rectum, pale face; especially for pinworms
- Stannum 6C: Pale sunken eyes with blue rings sluggish bowels, fetid breath, passive fever, prefers to lie on stomach
- Sulphur 30C: Eruptions on the skin, sinking sensation in epigastrium in the forenoon, hot head, cold feet
- Tanacetum vulgare 6C: Lassitude, brain fatigue, dysentery, reflex spasms
- Terebintha 6C: Burning and crawling in the anus
- Teucrium Marum Verum 9C: Anal itching, itchy rectum and nose, itchiness worse in evening, child restless in sleep, complains of crawling sensation in rectum after passing stools, much irritation in the rectum, constant irritation in the evening when in bed; commonly prescribed for the roundworm, *Ascaris*.

Appendix A

HERBAL FORMULAS

The following are examples of products on the market that are used to treat parasites. None of these formulas should be used by pregnant or breast-feeding women. These formulations may be used alone or in combination with other supportive measures depending on the duration and severity of the infection. In more severe chronic intestinal parasitic infection rebuilding the intestinal mucosa and reestablishing healthy flora may be as important as eradicating the pathogenic organisms.

Professional Complementary Health Formulas

P.O. Box 80085, Portland, OR 97280-1085
(800) 952-2219

Available herbal formulas are Botanifuge and Herbalfuge. These products are provided in capsules for assured delivery to the bowel—Botanifuge to inhibit the growth of organisms, and Herbalfuge for the expulsion of the parasite. Their products are only sold to licensed health professionals. Contact your doctor for more information. They also have homeopathic parasite remedies available.

BOTANIFUGE

This product is recommended for people over the age of 12 years old. Take one capsule before each meal and at bedtime. One capsule contains:

Black walnut (*Juglans nigra*)75 mg.
Oregano (standardized extract)75 mg.
Quassia (*Picrasma excelsa* extract)75 mg.
Wormwood (*Artemesia annua*)50 mg.
Cloves (*Syzgium aromaticum*)50 mg.
Garlic (*Allium sativa* extract)50 mg.
Plantain (*Plantago major*)50 mg.
Pumpkin seed (*Cucubita pepo*)50 mg.
Barberry (*Berberis vulgaris*)25 mg.
Goldenseal (*Hydrastis canadensis*)25 mg.
Grapefruit seed extract25 mg.
Male fern (*Dryopteris filix-mas*)25 mg.

Undecylenic acid15 mg.
Berberine sulfate10 mg.
Fennel (*Foeniculum vulgare*)10 mg.
Gentian (*Gentiana lutea*)10 mg.

HERBALFUGE

This product comes in a base of alfalfa root, cranebill root, fenugreek seed, flaxseed, goldenseal, mullein leaves, myrrh gum, poke root, white oak bark, witch hazel bark at 5 mg. each. This product is recommended for people over the age of 12 years old. Take one capsule before each meal and at bedtime. One capsule contains:

Pink root (*Spigella marylandica*)130 mg.
Culvers root (*Leptandra virginica*) 65 mg.
Senna pods/leaves (Cassia) 65 mg.
Violet leaves (*Viola odorata*) 65 mg.
Cascara sagrada (*Rhamnus purshiana*) 32 mg.
Slippery elm root (*Ulmus fulva*) 32 mg.
Pomegranate (*Punica granatum*) 5 mg.

Metagenics Northwest

Microbex, Candicin, and Parex Intensive Care are specially formulated blends using selected herbs and herbal extracts that have traditionally been used to support the body's defense system and to support a healthy intestinal environment. Metagenics Northwest can be reached at (800) 338-3948 or fax them at (541) 345-0787. The following products are sold only to licensed health professionals. Have your doctor call for more information.

MICROBEX

It is recommended to take 2 tablets three times daily between meals. One tablet contains:

Old Man's Beard (*Usnea barbata*) 182 mg.
Grapefruit Seed Extract (*Citrus paradisi*) 100 mg.
Oregon Grape Root (*Mahonia aquifolia*) 75 mg.
Barberry (*Berberis vulgaris*) 50 mg.
Goldenseal Root (*Hydrastis canadensis*) 25 mg.
Cat's Claw Vine (*Uncaria tomentosa*) 25 mg.

PAREX INTENSIVE CARE
The recommended dosage is 2 tablets three times daily between meals. One tablet contains:

Ficin (*Ficus glabrata*) 2.5 mg
Artemisia Leaf (*Artemisia annua*)120 mg.
Oregon Grape Root (*Mahonia aquifolia*) 50 mg
Goldenseal Root (*Hydrastis canadensis*) 20 mg.
Barberry Root (*Berbersi vulgaris*) 50 mg.
Gentia Root (*Gentiana lutea*) 75 mg.
Plantain Leaf (*Plantago major*)100 mg.
Black Walnut Green Hull (*Juglans nigra*) 50 mg.
Pumpkin Seed (*Cucurbita pepo*)150 mg.

CANDICIN
The recommended dosage is 1-2 tablets three times daily between meals. One tablet contains:

Grapefruit Seed Extract (*Citrus paradisi*) 120 mg.
Black Walnut Hull (*Juglans nigra*) 100 mg.
Slippery Elm Bark (*Ulmus fulva*) 91 mg.
Goldenseal Root (*Hydrastis canadensis*) 80 mg.
Bearberry Leaf (*Artostaphylos uva ursi*) 50 mg.

Tyler Encapsulations
The following formula contains substances and their dosage that have been helpful in the treatment of protozoa, especially *Entamoeba histolytica, Giardia lamblia, Trichomonas vaginalis*, and others, such as the chlorquine-resistant protozoa found in malaria. The following product is only sold to licensed healthcare professionals. Have your doctor call them toll-free for product information or consult with one of their staff physicians at (800) 869-9705. Contact them on the internet at www.tyler-inc.com.

PARA-GARD
The general dosage directions are 2-3 capsules three times daily on an empty stomach or inbetween meals or as directed by your physician. Child dosage is 1 cap 2-3 times a day. Do not use during pregnancy, lactation, and active liver disease. They have a 4-8 week protocol starting with establishing adequate digestion two weeks before taking the parasite medication. One capsule contains:

Berberine sulfate 100 mg.
Grapefruit Seed extract 100 mg.
Gentiana lutea extract (gentian) 4:1 concentrate75 mg.
Hydrastis canadensis extract (goldenseal) 5 percent
Hydrastine 50 mg.
Artemesia annua (Chinese wormwood) 50 mg.
Picrasma excelsa extract (quassia) 50 mg.
Juglans nigra extract (black walnut hull) 50 mg.
Allium sativa extract (garlic) 0.8 percent Allicin 50 mg.

Appendix B

USING DRUGS TO TREAT PARASITES

Progress and technology has made our world a better place, but it may not have made it safer. Medical science has been at least partly responsible for bringing about this situation and can we depend on them to get us out of this problem? Will a pharmacologically-based medical system develop new and stronger drugs? The overuse of drugs is part of the problem of producing superbugs. It would seen reasonable to seek other methods and approaches to protect our health if possible.

Sometimes the better choice in cases of severe or life-threatening parasitic infections is to use prescription drugs. Antiparasitic prescription drugs should also be considered for people who do not respond to more natural therapies. Even people who have had chronic, resistant cases should not be discouraged, but consult with their doctors, as they can probably benefit from some of the new drug treatments. Drug therapy is often recommended, because it is rapid and fairly sure. Dietary treatment for these conditions are much slower, but the role of diet and nutritional factors should be helpful in preventing reinfection or as a supportive measure even when using drug treatment.

When antibiotics and other drugs are used to treat parasites, they can pose a threat to the overall health of a person by disturbing the natural balance of the body's own immune system. This is especially true for people with an already compromised immune system or those who are chronically ill. Most drugs are toxic and should not be taken over an extended period. Since many parasites need to be treated for long periods, the use of drugs can themselves cause many problems. The need to use drugs must be weighed against how toxic the drug is. Some of these drugs can cause severe side effects. Sometimes it is better to take a lesser effective drugs for a longer period than choose the more effective and toxic one. Consult your physician for prescriptions and dose schedules.

In many cases, antiparasitic prescriptive drugs have not proven to be effective. The symptoms may decrease for a couple of months and later return. Many people take several different types of medications, and no one is concerned how they will affect the parasites in the body. One unknown side effect of drugs is that they can drive a parasite from one organ to another. Worms can wander out of their normal environment in the body when they encounter adverse conditions. A typical example is the finding of *Ascaris* in the bile duct or liver. These worms do not commonly leave the intestinal tract unless the patient takes a drug that is toxic, but not lethal to the parasite, or unless there happens to be a gastro-intestinal disorder that alters the normal digestive process.

This shows a potential danger of drugs that most doctors are not aware of. Imagine if a person takes a drug to eliminate one problem and this drug indirectly drives a parasite from its natural resting place into another organ such as the liver. If the person later comes down with severe liver problems, no one will ever know what caused the problem in the first place. I strongly recommend you see a health professional trained to guide you in the treatment of parasites, because you do not want the cure to be worse than the parasitic infection.

Some of the organisms I have discussed in this book were not considered pathogens even a few years ago, but today they are. This makes the elimination of parasites more difficult than in the past. One of the reasons is that parasites are becoming resistant to many of the prescription drugs that are used to kill them. Drugs such as quinacrine, megendazole, and medtronidazole are losing their effectiveness. In the past a doctor could give a single course of these drugs and it would be effective against most cases of protozoa infections, but not today. Often, these toxic drugs have to be taken for long periods. This is what makes them so harmful to the body and produces undesirable side effects. Because of the long life cycle of many parasites, it can take three months to eradicate them. This is why a comprehensive holistic approach is usually the most desirable rather than just prescription drugs alone.

Appendix C

RULES FOR DOSING CHILDREN AND THE ELDERLY WITH HERBAL MEDICATION

Most herbal products give dosage based on people who weigh 150 lbs. There is a need to scale up or down for those who weight a lot less or more, taking into consideration present and inherent vitality.

1. Children's Dose

- Clark's Rule is the most commonly used formula for dosing children. Find out the child's weight in pounds and divide by 150 pounds. This equals the fraction of adult dose used.

- King's American Dispensary uses the following doses for children:

    6 months or younger = 1/15 of the adult dose
    1 year: 1/12 of the adult dose
    2 years: 1/8 of the adult dose
    3 years: 1/6 of the adult dose
    4 years: 1/5 of the adult dose
    7 years: 1/3 of the adult dose
    14 years: 1/2 of the adult dose
    20 years: 2/3 of the adult dose

2. The Elderly's Dose

- Basing the dose on the weight and strength of the person is the best method. Make sure the patient is well hydrated, directions on how to take the medication is well understood, knowing what other medications are being taken, and how any interaction of the medicines could effect the patient. The digestive system should be in reasonably good order. One of the accepted guidelines recommends to reduce the adult dose by 1/4 for persons over 65; reduce by 1/2 for those over 70. The dose can vary depending on the general health of the person being treated. These are only guidelines; each case should be evaluated individually for the best results.

• Another guideline for adjusting dosage for the age of the person is when the adult dose is one teaspoonful based on 60 grains or drops:

Children 3 months old or less: 2 grains/drops
Children from 3 to 6 months: 3
Children from 6 to 9 months: 4
Children from 9 to 12 months: 5
Children from 12 to 18 months: 7
Children from 18 to 24 months: 8
Children from 2 to 3 years: 10
Children from 3 to 4 years: 12
Children from 4 to 6 years: 15
Children from 6 to 9 years: 24
Children from 9 to 12 years: 30
Children from 12 to 15 years: 38
Children from 15 to 18 years: 45
Anyone from 18 to 21 years: 60 grains/drops

• When the adult dose is one teacup:

Children one year old or less: 2 teaspoonsful
Children from 2 to 4 years old: 3
Children from 4 to 7 years old: 1 tablespoonful
Children from 7 to 11 years old: 2
Children from 11 to 15 years old: 3
Children from 15 to 18 years old: 4
Youths from 18 to 21 years old: 5
Anyone 21 years old and over: 1 teacup

• Powders either mixed in water or in capsules when the adult dose is one dram based on 1 dram = 1 teaspoon or 60 grains:

Children one year or less: 33 grains
Children from 1 to 2 years: 6 grains
Children from 2 to 3 years: 9 grains
Children from 3 to 4 years: 12 grains
Children from 4 to 8 years: 18 grains
Children from 8 to 13 years: 25 grains
Children from 13 to 18 years: 40 grains
Youths from 18 to 21 years: 60 grains

Resources

Travel
- You can obtain information from the Traveler's Medical Service of Washington, DC., by calling them at (202) 466-8109 for pretravel information on food, water, and other hygienic practices.
- Contact the Traveler's Health Section of the Centers for Disease Control in "Atlanta (404) 639-3311 to get a guide to the regional diseases in the areas where you will be going.

Acquiring Drugs To Treat Parasites
- CDC Drug Service, Centers for Disease Control, Atlanta, Georgia 30333, (404) 639-3670. Some drugs used to fight parasites are available for your physician from the CDC.
- The National Institute of Allergy and Infectious Diseases has available to your physician some of the drugs used to treat parasites. Contact them at (800) 537-9978.

Physician Referral
There are many sources to find out about a naturopathic physician in your area. You could look in your phone directory under "physicians, naturopathic," or ask at your local health food store for a referral. Check with other healthcare professionals in your area such as your chiropractor. You can also contact our national association to see who is in your area and about their expertise:

American Association of Naturopathic Medicine
601 Valley Street, Suite 105
Seattle, WA 98109
Phone: (206) 298-0126 Fax: (206) 298-0125

Call them for a referral to a naturopathic physician in your area. They are the only licensed physicians who are trained in colon therapy in medical school. They are also well trained to use herbal medicine, homeopathy, and nutrition in the treatment of disease.

Consultations
Dr. Skye Weintraub, ND
911 Country Club Rd., Suite 300
Eugene, OR 97401
(541) 345-0747 or contact me by E-mail at drskye@aol.com.

I will be available to consult with you about the information you have read in this book concerning parasites. Call to set up a time by phone. Hopefully, by the time you read this book, I will also have a web site available that will provide even more information about parasites and their treatment.

Dr. F. Russell Manuel, M.D., MSc.
Wholestic Research Group
P.O. box 95, Lummi Island, WA 98262
voice mail (888) WHOLE44

Dr. Manuel is a holistic medical consultant who gives lectures and seminars. He also provides information and consultations to individuals and health professionals. Ask for a catalogue of printed materials, books, audios, and videos.

Colonic Therapists
Contact one of these associations to find a colonic therapist in your area:

California Colon Hygienists Society
PO Box 588
Graton, CA 95444
(707) 829-0984
Refers to a nationwide network of colon therapists.

International Association for Colon Therapy
2051 Hilltop Drive, Suite A-11
Redding, CA 96002
(916) 222-1498
Refers to a nationwide network of colon therapists.

Wood Hygienic Institute, Inc.
PO Box 420580
Kissimmee, FL 34742
(407) 933-0009
Refers practitioners in colon therapy.

Parasitology OnLine
http://www.paru.cas.cz/parasito.htm
A web site that will link you with many other sites that deal with the subject of parasites.

Parasite Searches
http://www.ncbi.nlm.nih.gov/htbin-post/Entrez/query?db=m&form=0
http://www.healthgate.com/HealthGate/MEDLINE/search.shtml

Parasitology Pages
http://www-personal.ksu.edu/~coccidia/
http://martin.parasitology.mcgill.ca/JIMSPAGE/WORLDOF.HTM
http://dspace.dial.pipex.com/town/plaza/aan18/urls.htm
http://www-museum.unl.edu/asp_image/links.html

Parasitology Journals
http://www.uniduesseldorf.de/WWW/MathNat/Parasitologie/para_jou.htm

The following are some of the journals available online for the further study of parasites:

- *Advances in Parasitology*
- *American Journal of Tropical Medicine and Hygiene*
- *Annals of Tropical Medicine and Parasitology*
- *Current Advances in Immunology and Infectious Disease*
- *Epidemiology and Infection*
- *Helminthological Abstracts*
- *International Journal for Parasitology*
- *Internet Journal of Parasitology*
- *Journal of Helminthology*
- *Journal of Infectious Diseases*
- *Journal of Parasitology*
- *Malaria Weekly*
- *Parasitology International*
- *Parasitology Research*
- *Parasitology Today*
- *Protozoological Abstracts*
- *Tropical Medicine and International Health*
- *Veterinary Parasitology*

References From Books

Barney, Paul. *Clinical Applications of Herbal Medicine.* UT: Woodland Pub, UT: 1996.

Beneson, Abram S. *Control of Communicable Diseases in Man.* Washington DC: American Public Health Association, 1985.

Bolyard, Judith. *Medicinal Plants and Home Remedies of Appalachia.* IL: Charles C. Thomas Pub, 1981.

Buchman, Dian Dincin. *Herbal Medicine-The Natural Way to Get Well and Stay Well.* NY: Gramercy Pub, 1979.

Burton Goldberg Group. *Alternative Medicine.* WA: Future Medicine Pub, 1995.

Clark, Hulda R. *The Cure for all Cancers.* CA: New Centruy Press, 1993.

Clarke, John Henry. *The Prescriber.* England: Health Science Press, 1983.

Coon, Nelson. *Using Plants for Healing.* PA: Rodale Press, 1979.

DeSchepper, Luc. *Peak Immunity.* CA: L. DeSchepper, 1990.

Gittleman, Louise A. *Guess What Came To Dinner.* NY; Avery Pub, 1993.

Griffin, LaDean. *Please Doctor, I'd Rather Do It Myself with Herbs!* UT: Hawkes Pub, 1979.

Griffin, LaDean. *Is any Sick Among You?* UT: Bi-World Pub, 1982.

Heinerman, John. *Science of Herbal Medicine.* UT: Bi-World Pub, 1979.

Holmes, Peter. *Energetics of Western Herbs.* CO: Artemis Press, 1989.

Hutchens, Elam R. *Indian Herbalogy of North America.* 1973.

Kadans, Joseph. *Encyclopedia of Medicinal Herbs.* NY: Arco Pub, 1980.

Kent, JT. *Repertory of the Homeopathic Materia Medica.* New Delhi: Jain Pub, 1984.

Kroeger, Hanna. *Parasites-The Enemy Within.* CO: Hanna Kroeger Publications, 1991.

Miller, Benjamin F. *The Complete Medical Guide.* NY: Simon and Schuster, 1978.

Moore, Michael. *Medicinal Plants of the Mountain West.* NM: The Museum of New Mexico Press, 1979.

Krupp, Marcus A, Lawrence M. Tierney, et al. *Physician's Handbook— Twenty-First Edition.* CA: Lange Medical Pub, 1985.

Lewis, Walter H. *Medical Botany.* NY: John Wiley & Sons, 1977.

Ritchason, Jack. *The Little Herb Encyclopedia.* UT: Woodland Health Books, 1995.

Royal, Penny C. *Herbally Yours.* UT: BiWorld Pub,1981.

Schnurrenberger, Paul R, Hubbert, William T. *An Outline of the Zoonoses.* IA: Iowa State University Press, 1981.

Sharamon, Shalila, Baginski, Bodo J. *The Healing Power of Grapefruit Seed.*

WI: Lotus Light Pub, 1996.

Shook, Edward. *Elementary Treatise in Herbology*. CA: Trinity Center Press, 1974.

Spizizen, John. *Medical Microbiology*. NY: Elsevier Science Pub, 1984.

Tenney, Louise. *Today's Herbal Health*. UT: Hawthorne Books, 1982.

Tenney, Louise. *Today's Herbal Health for Children*. UT: Woodland Pub, 1996.

Thrash, Agatha, Thrash, Calvin. *Home Remedies*. AL: Thrash Pub, 1981.

Tierra, Michael. *The Way of Herbs*. NY: Washington Square Press, 1983.

Trattler, Ross. *Better Health Through Natural Healing*. NY: McGraw-Hill, 1985.

Treben, Maria. *Health Through God's Pharmacy*. Austria: Wilhelm Ennsthaler Pub, 1983.

Treben, Maria. *Health from God's Garden*. VT: Healing Arts Press, 1988.

References From Journals

Amin, Omar M. "Prevalence and Host Relationships of Intestinal Protozoan Infections During the Summer of 1996," *Explore* 8(1997):29-35.

Archer, Douglas L, Walter H. Glinsmann, "Enteric Infection and Other Cofactors in AIDS," *Immunology Today* 9(1985).

Bhakat, MP, Nandi N, et al. "Therapeutic Trial of Berberine Sulfate in Non-specific Gastroenteritis," *Ind Med J* 68(1974):19-23.

Birdsall, Timothy C, Kelly, Gregory S. "Berberine: Therapeutic Potential of an Alkaloid Found in Several Medicinal Plants," *Alt Med Rev* 2(2)(1997):94-103.

Borst, P, et al. "Antigenic Variation in Malaria," *Cell* 82(1995):1-4.

Brown, EAE. et al. "Cryptosporidiosis in Great Yarmouth-The Investigation Of An Outbreak," *Public Health* 103(1989):3-9.

Burke, TM, Roberson, EL. "Prenatal and Lactational Transmission of Toxocara canis and Ancyclostoma caninum: Experimental Infection of the Bitch BeforePregnancy," *Int J Parasitol* 15(1985):71-75.

Canning, EU. "Parasitic and Other Infections in AIDS," *Transactions of the Royal Society of Tropical Medicine and Hygiene* 84(1990):19-24.

Casemore, DP. "Epidemiological Aspects of Human Cryptosporidiosis," *Epidemiology and Infection* 104(1990):1-28.

Choudhry, VP, et al. "Berberine in Giardiasis," *Indian Pediatrics* 9(3)(1972):143-146.

Clancy, JL, et al. "Commercial Labs: How Accurate Are They? " *Jour Am Water Works Assoc* 86(1994):89-97.

Clark, Alice M, et al. "Antimicrobial Activity of Juglone," *Phytotherapy Research* 4(1990):11.

Current, WL "The Biology of Cryptosporidium," *ASM News* 54(1988): 605-611.

Current, WL;, et al. "Human Cryptosporidiosis in Immunocompetent and Immunodeficient Persons. Studies of an Putbreak and Experimental Transmission," *New Eng Jour of Med* 308(1983):1252-1257.

Current, WL, Garcia, LS. "Cryptosporidiosis," *Clinical Microbiology Reviews* 4(1991): 325-358.

Current, WL, Reese, NC. "A Comparison of Endogenous Development of Three Isolates of Cryptosporidium in Suckling Mice," *Journal of Protozoology* 33(1986):98-108.

Current, WL, Upton, SJ, et al. "The Life Cycle of Cryptosporidium Infecting Chickens," *Journal of Protozoology* 33(1986):289- 296.

D'Antonio, RG, et al. "A Waterborne Outbreak of Cryptosporidiosis in Normal Hosts," *Annals of Internal Medicine* 103(1985):886-888.

Dubey, JP, Speer, CA, et al."Cryptosporidiosis of Man and Animals," *CRC Press* (1990):199.

Fayer, R, Ungar, BLP. 1986. "Cryptosporidium spp. and Cryptosporidiosis. *Microbiological Reviews* 50(1986):458-483.

Fulzele, DP, Sipahimalani, AT, Heble, MR. "Tissue Cultures of Artemesia annua: Organogenesis and Artemesin Production," *Phytotherapy Res* 5(1991):149-153.

Gallaher, MM, et al. "Cryptosporidiosis and Surface Water," *Amer Jour of Pub Health* 79(1989):39-42.

Garavelli, PL, Scaglione, L, et al. "Blastocystosis: A New Disease in Patients With Leukemia," *Haematologica* (1991):76:80.

Garavelli, Pl, et al. "Blastocystosis: A New Disease in the Acquired Immunodeficiency Syndrome?" *Int J STD AIDS* 1(1990):134-135.

Garcia, LS, Bruckner, Da, et al. "Clinical Relevance of Blastocystis hominis," *Lancet* 1(1984):1233-1234.

Glickman, LT, Schantz, PM. "Epidemiology and Pathogenesis of Zoonotic Toxocariasis," *Epidemiol Rev* 3(1981);230-250.

Haynes, EB, et al. "Large Community Outbreak of Cryptosporidiosis Due to Contamination of a Filtered Public Water Supply," *New Eng Jour of Med* 320(1989):1372-1376.

Hughs, BG, Lawson, LD. "Antimicrobial Effects of Allium sativum (garlic), Allium ampeloprasm (elephant garlic), and Allium cepa (onion), Garlic Compounds and Commercial Garlic Supplement Products," *Phytother Res* 5(1991):154-158.

Hunninghake, Ronald E. "Comparison of Two Methods of Intestinal Parasite Detection," *Townsend Letter for Doctors* (1992):956.

Ionescuy, F, et al, "Oral Citrus Seed Extract in Atopic Excema: In Vitro and in Vivo Studies on Intestinal Microflora," *J Ortho Med* 5(3)(1990): 155-8.

Joseph, C. et al. "Cryptosporidiosis in the Isle of Thanet; An Outbreak Associated with Local Drinking Water," *Epidemiology and Infection* 107(1991):509-519.

Kalkofen, VP. "Hookworms of Dogs and Cats," *Vet Clin North Am Small Anim Pract* 17(1987);1341-1354.

Kaneda, Y, Torii, M, et al. "In Vitro Effects of Berberine Sulfate on the Growth and Structure of Entamoeba histolytica, Giardia lamblia and Trichomonas vaginalis," *Ann Trop Med Parasit* 85(4)(1991):417-425.

Kent, GP, et al. "Epidemic Giardiasis Caused by a Contaminated Public Water Supply," *AJPH* 78(2)(1988).

Kirby, GC, O'Neill, MJ, et al, "In Vitro Studies on the Mode of Action of Quassinoids With Activity Against Chloroquine-Resistant Plasmodium falciparum," *Biochem Pharm* 389(24)(1989):4367-4374.

Koberla, F. "Chagas Disease and Chagas' Syndromes:the Pathology of American Trypanosomiasis," *Advances in Parasitology* 6(1988):63-116.

Lee, Martin J. "Parasites, Yeasts and Bacteria in Health and Disease," *Jour Adv Med* 8(2)(1995):121-129.

LeLand, D, et al. "A Cryptosporidiosis Outbreak in a Filtered-Water Supply," *Journal of the American Water Works Association* 85(1993):34-42.

Lisle, JT,Rose, JB. "Cryptosporidium Contamination of Water in the USA and UK: A Mini-Review," *J. Water SRT-Aqua* 44(1995):103-117.

MacKenzie, WR, et al. "Massive Outbreak of Waterborne Cryptosporidium Infection in Milwaukee, Wisconsin. Recurrence of Illness and Risk of Secondary Transmission," *Clin Inf Dis* 21(1995):57-62.

MacKenzie, WR, et al. "A Massive Outbreak in Milwaukee of Cryptosporidium Infection Transmitted Through the Public Water Supply," *New Eng Jour of Med* 331(1994):161-167.

Millard, PS, et al. "An Outbreak of Cryptosporidiosis From Fresh-Pressed Apple Cider," *Jour of the Amer Med Assoc* 272(1994):1592-1596.

Mirelman, D, Monheit, D, Varon, S, "Inhibition of Growth of Entamoeba histolytica by Allicin, The Active Principle of Garlic Extract (Allium sativum)," *J Inf Dis* 156(1) (1987):243-244.

Murray, Michael T. "Ginger (Zingiber Officinale)," *Amer J Nat Med* 3(7)(1996):12-16.

Murray, Michael T. "Curcumin: A potent anti-inflammatory agent," *Amer J Nat Med* 12(4)(1994):10-13.

Murray, Michael T. "Traveler's Diarrhea: The Benefits of Plants Containing Berberine," *Phyto-Pharmica Review* 3(3)(1990):3-4.

Newswire. "Parasitic Disease Found Among Gulf Vets," *Townsend Letter for Doctors* 7(1992):628-629.

Nguyen, De, Dao, BH, et al. "Treatment of Malaria in Vietnam With Oral Artemesinin," *Am J Trop Med Hyg* 48(3)(1993):398-40.

O'Donoghue, PJ. "Cryptosporidium and Cryptosporidiosis in Man and Animals," *International Jour for Parasitology* 25(1995):139-195.

Parsons, JC. "Ascarid Infections in Cats and Dogs," *Vet Clin North Am Small Anim Pract* 17(1987):1307-1339.

Pearce, Richard B. "Intestinal Protozoal Infections and AIDS," *Lancet* (1983).

Phillipson, J. David, Wright, Colin W. "Medicinal Plants in Tropical Medicine," *Royal Society of Tropical Medicine and Hygiene Meeting at Manson House,* London (1990):29-39.

Rasmussen, KR, Healey, MC. "Dehydroepiandrosterone-Induced Reduction of Cryptosporidium parvum Infections in Aged Syrian Golden Hamsters," *J Parasitology* 78 (1992):554-556.

Ricci, N, Toma, P, et al. "Blastocystis hominis: A Neglected Cause of Diarrhea?" *Lancet* 1 (1984);966.

Ronzio, Robert A. "Antioxidants, Nutraceuticals and Functional Foods," *Townsend Letter for Doctors* (1997):34.

Smith, HV, Rose, JB. "Waterborne Cryptosporidiosis," *Parasitology Today* 6(1990):8-12.

Steinberg, Phillip N. "Cat's Claw Update," *Townsend Letter for Doctors* (1995):70.

Sweryzcek, TW, Nielsen, SW, Helmbolt, CF. "Transmammary Passage of Toxocara cati in the Cat," *Am J Vet Res* 32(1971);89-92.

Tzipori, S. "Cryptosporidiosis of Animals and Humans," *Microbiological Reviews* 47 (1983):84-96.

Walker, Morton. "You Can Eliminate Parasites to Cure All Diseases," *Townsend Letter for Doctors* 2(1997):64-70.

Zagury, D, et al. "Long-term Cultures of HTLV-III-infected T- cells: A Model of Cytopathology of T-cell Depletion in AIDS," *Science* (1986).

Index